To the Seventh Generation

The Journey of Christian Medical College Vellore

Dr. V I Mathan

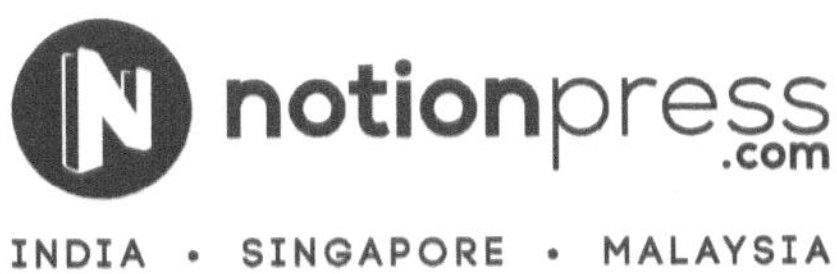

INDIA · SINGAPORE · MALAYSIA

ISBN
Paperback 979-8-89610-679-1
Hardcase 979-8-89673-799-5

Contents

Foreword

With immense pleasure and a deep sense of responsibility, I pen this foreword for "To the Seventh Generation" by Dr. VI Mathan. This book is a testament to the enduring legacy of the Christian Medical College, Vellore (CMCV). This legacy is deeply rooted in our commitment to medical excellence and compassionate care. For over a century, this Institution has been a beacon of these values, and this commitment guides us in our journey forward.

One must know, where one came from to direct one's path forward. This applies as much to institutions as it does to individuals. There should be no scope for dilution of the founding principles, and for this, a clear understanding of all that went to define it, the immense sacrifices that were made, and the difficult decisions that were taken need to be understood and contextualised so that subsequent generations learn to value and cherish what they possess. Understanding our past, is not just about preserving history but about learning from it, drawing inspiration from the struggles and triumphs of those who came before us, and using that knowledge to shape a better future.

I can think of no better person to chronicle the accurate history of the evolution of CMCV and to describe its birth pangs, tumultuous growth, and current stature than Dr. VI Mathan. Dr. Mathan was in the last generation who had direct personal contact with our founder.Having a personal communication, I know that he was deeply influenced by her and promised her to dedicate his life to the Institution. He has done this in his lifetime of service in various capacities as a student, faculty member, and multiple administrative roles over the years, and after retirement, a regular attendee at every council meeting as an ex– director. No one has seen up– close the working and evolution of this Institution as much as Dr. Mathan has.

Since its inception in 1900 by Dr. Ida Sophia Scudder, CMCV has been driven by a singular ethos: to serve humanity with the utmost dedication, humility, and love. The history of CMCV is a chronicle of individuals and the Institution surpassing immense challenges. From the early days of setting up the Mary Taber Schell Hospital to navigating the complex socio–political landscapes of a newly independent India, it faced an existential crisis with forces inimical to its existence and many more. The Institution's ability to adapt and grow in response to these challenges is a testament to the resilience and foresight of its leaders and faculty. Each generation of students and staff has contributed to this growth, ensuring that CMCV remains at the forefront of medical education and healthcare. This narrative book highlights that at the heart of CMCV's success is its community. Driven by a common purpose, the faculty, staff, and students work harmoniously. This sense of community, which we are all a part of, distinguishes CMCV from many other institutions. It fosters an environment where knowledge is imparted, shared, and nurtured. The collaborative spirit, the commitment to excellence, honesty, integrity, and the unwavering dedication to service are the cornerstones of CMCV's ethos.

Dr. Mathan's book delves deep into the contributions of key figures who have shaped CMCV. From the early pioneers who worked alongside Dr. Scudder to the current generation of leaders, each has been crucial in steering the Institution toward greater heights. The detailed accounts of their efforts provide invaluable insights into the factors contributing to CMCV's sustained excellence.

As we move further into the 21st century, medical education and healthcare challenges are evolving; the rapid advancements in medical science and technology and the increasing commercialisation of healthcare present new hurdles that we are forced to deal with. Yet, CMCV continues to uphold its founding principles, adapting to modern demands while staying true to its core values. This balance between tradition and innovation will guide CMCV through the coming decades.

To the Seventh Generation is more than just a historical account; it is a source of inspiration and a call to action. It reminds us of the importance of service, the power of community, and the enduring legacy of those who came before us. Dr. Mathan's meticulous documentation and heartfelt narratives provide a comprehensive understanding of CMCV's journey and its place in the annals of medical history. This book is also a must-read for all administrators, present and future; all administrations make errors, but to repeat historical errors is not pardonable. The need for the administration and administrators to be strong, resilient, and decisive and not pander to or appease individuals or forces that are not in the Institution's interest in the short and long–term, is critical. This can be at the expense of personal popularity and may come at a high cost.

However, the institution is always above individuals, and the consequences of failure to do so are illustrated well in this book. The book also documents the evolution of many of our governing principles and existing administrative structures and manuals, with in–built checks and balances demonstrating our predecessors' wisdom, foresight, and dedication. These processes and systems have stood us in good stead over the years.

As we look to the future, may we continue to be guided by the principles that have defined CMCV for over a century. May we strive to uphold the legacy of Dr. Ida Sophia Scudder and ensure that the spirit of service, compassion, and excellence continues to shine brightly for generations to come.

With heartfelt gratitude and admiration

Dr. Vikram Mathews MD, DM FASc
Director, Christian Medical College, Vellore

Preface

The continued growth and development of the Christian Medical College, Vellore (CMCV) has prompted those involved or interested in the Institution to ask three questions:

Many institutions founded by charismatic, dynamic and totally dedicated individuals driven by their vision, falter and wither within two to three decades of their death. This has not happened to CMCV–Why?

Patients usually seek big–name doctors especially when they are looking for a court of last resort for their ailments. Why do the majority of patients who come to CMCV come to this Institution and not look for a specified big–name doctor?

Doctors are egotistical and compete with each other and are keenly interested in their own glory. Why do the faculty at Vellore, work in relative harmony and cooperate with each other, to train the large student body for the benefit of the patients who seek help at CMCV?

This Institution was founded in 1900 by a lady Doctor, Ida Sophia Scudder, a citizen of the United States of America, born in India 30 years earlier, to missionary parents. When she was first taken back to the United States of America at the age of seven, after she had seen the ravages of the Great Famine of 1887 as an impressionable child, she vowed that she would never come back to this dirty, filthy land of poverty. This decision was further strengthened during her studies in the US. However, she came back 23 years later, driven by a passion, to improve the health of the women and children of India, a passion that changed to a conviction that drove her to train Indian women to help their sisters and children? Why are we still driven by her dreams, 60 years after her death?

The answer given rather glibly by many, at CMCV is 'It is our ethos'. What is ethos? The Oxford Dictionary defines 'ethos' as "characteristic spirit or attitude of a community". Anyone who spends time at CMCV will see that it functions as a community. The ethos of CMCV ensures concern, care and honesty to the patient, a fellow creation of God. To serve a fellow human, is an opportunity to express God's love through the knowledge and skills He has vested in you. How has this ethos evolved during the 120 years of CMCV?

I joined this community as a first–year medical student almost 70 years ago in 1955, when Dr. Ida Sophia Scudder, known to all her students and colleagues as 'Aunt Ida', was very much a living presence in the community. My wife and I were privileged as students to interact with her on the campus and be influenced by the spirit she infused into all who came in contact with her and the community,at large. Most of our teachers, were her colleagues or students and they nurtured us in the spirit embodied in our motto: "Not to be ministered unto, but to minister".

The death of the founder of an institution, is a cataclysmic trauma and the Christian Medical College Vellore experienced this in May 1960. It was fortunate that in 1960 there were many in the Institution who had worked for long with the founder, not only as a faculty but also as staff of all categories who had been inspired by her in person and who could continue to build on her vision. Forty years later, in 2000, the Centenary year of the Institution, the staff and faculty who had known Aunt Ida in person, had retired. Currently, there is no one who knew Aunt Ida personally working at Vellore, but a few retired staff who are still around, who have vivid and valued memories of their interactions with her.

There are three books which are a must to understand the significant contributions of the Scudder family and the life and witness of Aunt Ida.

A Thousand Years in Thy Sight is a detailed account of the Scudder families' contributions to India, written by Dorothy J Scudder, the wife of Dr. John Scudder III, the great–grandson of Dr. John Scudder, who started the Scudder saga in India in 1819. John III, the son of Aunt Ida's brother, worked at the Scudder Memorial Hospital, Ranipet from 1929 to 1935 and his wife researched and wrote this book after their return to the USA during the latter half of the 1940's. It was first published in 1970 privately and with added photographs was republished in 1984 by the Vantage Press. The second book was written by Dr. Mary Pauline Jeffrey, who was inspired by Aunt Ida and who changed her profession from a missionary teacher to a doctor. In this, she was helped by Gertrude Dodd, a companion of Aunt Ida for decades and whose financial support ensured the survival of the Institution at critical points. Pauline Jeffrey worked at Vellore and later founded the Kotagiri Medical Fellowship. She wrote *Ida S Scudder of Vellore* in 1934, which was updated and republished in 1980 titled *Passing on the Torch of Life*. There are also a number of books by or on the lives and contributions of many faculty who joined CMCV after Aunt Ida had made the hard decision to change the Missionary Medical School for Women to a coeducational Medical College. While these books help us to understand the contributions of the Scudder family and others, and the wonderful life of Aunt Ida, none of them attempted a history of CMCV. To answer the three questions posed at the beginning, we have to travel the long journey of the last 120 years.

The material available at Vellore till 1920 is very limited. But after that, the minutes of the meetings of the Governing Council and the reports of the Principal, the Director and other Administrative officers documented the growth and development of CMC. This book is an attempt to analyse the available material, summarise the contributions of several of the key players in the development of CMCV and also to try and find the answers to the questions posed above.It is also to summarise the challenges faced by the Institution over the years and how they were faced and solved. It is not a biography of Aunt Ida but an attempt to identify and document the ethos of this Institution by one who has been privileged to be involved with CMCV since 1955. It is an attempt to be objective, as far as the facts are concerned but the analysis is coloured by my deep commitment to the Institution.

An institution can be divided into several generations usually starting with the founder. This book describes the generations that have gone into the making of the Christian Medical College, Vellore. The photographs at the end of the book provide a glimpse of some moments etched in history. Some are from my personal collection and some have been used with permission from the CMCV archives.

The story starts with Aunt Ida's grandparents in 1819 and goes forward with her parents and succeeding generation. Together, they contributed almost 100 years of service to India. It comes to the twenty–first century in the Seventh Generation who did not have the privilege or chance to know the founder in person. My wife and I were privileged to be of the Fifth Generation and trained as students when Aunt Ida was an inspiring presence on the campus, worked with the Sixth Generation and are now in a position to challenge the Seventh Generation. Let us understand and learn from the generations to inspire the Seventh Generation in the twenty–first century and the new millennium and more generations to come.

Dr. V I Mathan

Acknowledgements

I would like to acknowledge the many friends, too numerous to name, who prodded me to write the memoirs. It has been an enjoyable experience reminiscing and revisiting the past.

This book would not have been started by me except for the persistence of my daughter Anila and my son-in-law Anand Vurgese, who were more convinced than me that these jottings were very valuable. The companionship of my granddaughter Annika was refreshing and stimulating while writing.

A special name to be mentioned here is Sunttosh NM, a close friend of Anand, He was instrumental in introducing two friends from the publishing industry, Abrar and Jyotsna, who contributed significantly to the book in many ways. Abrar and Jyotsna engaged with me over conversational sittings to add final tweaks to the manuscript. Through diligent engagement, they helped transform the base manuscript into a fully packaged book. Additionally, Abrar worked closely with my family to finalise Notion Press to publish and market the book. I would also like to thank my son-in-law's close friend, Vikram Chesetty, for introducing us to Notion Press

To my friends and colleagues, Joyce Ponnaiya, Suranjan Bhattacharjee, Punnoose Mathew and Jasper Daniel, a big thank you for encouraging me to write and critically reviewing the manuscript. Special thanks to Punnoose for editing the document, both factually and grammatically. I thank Dr. Suresh David for the photograph used on the cover, Dr. Reena George for the photographs from CMCV archives, and Dr. Merlyn Fernando for the photographs of the 1955 Batch. I am also grateful to the present Director of CMCV, Prof. Vikram Mathews for his gracious foreword.

I would like to thank our family friend Mrs. Chitra Joseph for going out of her way and helping us with the "Final Editing" of the book and helping in the "Completion" of the book. I would like to thank my Son-in-Law's school mate Ashok Thomas and his wife Anitha Thomas for helping us with the book launch.

Finally, to my wife Minnie, not only for being by my side but also for doing much of the hard work of putting the book together. She has been and continues to be a constant support not only throughout the writing of the book but also throughout my life.

Introduction

Seven generations and more to come

The challenge of change is constant in life, requiring responses from individuals and institutions. The relevance of the response to this challenge can bring about dramatic changes in institutions, organisations and individuals. 2018 was the Centenary year of medical education at CMCV. We thank and praise God for the wonderful ways in which He has challenged and guided many to bring the Christian Medical College Vellore to 2018. It is worthwhile to pause and look back to our true beginning, learn from our history and discern the wonderful ways in which God brought us where we are. There were dark valleys and many shining peaks, as individuals were called and responded to challenges to follow the path He revealed each and every step of our journey.. Such reflection illuminates the way forward, may be only for the next day, the next week, the next month or the next year, till the challenge of change again catches up. It is sufficient to see only the next step clearly in our journey through medical education, for the next century and more of witnessing for the Kingdom of God.

The Christian Medical College Vellore (CMCV) now is a blend of its heritage, traditions and unique practices, influenced and modified by the changes and challenges in the society over the last century and more. It survives in a world very different from what confronted Dr. Ida Sophia Scudder ('Aunt Ida' to all her students) when she started her work in 1900, in Colonial India with its limited finance, transportation, communication and education. Events and changes caught up with Aunt Ida in her work at Vellore, forcing her to respond to changes even before independence from colonial rule in 1947, creating cataclysmic changes in the socioeconomic and political sphere. This was preceded in 1942 by the Quit India Movement, traumatic for (note the huge space) all foreign missionaries. The change of ownership of CMCV in 1955, from The Vellore Board in New York and other overseas missionary bodies to the Christian Medical College Vellore Association, a wholly Indian owned entity, was a dramatic transformation that was foreseen by Aunt Ida in 1942 and shepherded by her. The changes in India and the world in the seven decades since 1955 are even more striking. The art of medicine is now being transformed to the science and technology of medicine, progressing from intuitive care to evidence based protocols. Unfortunately, healthcare in the twenty–first century is seen as an industry, a very successful one, promising excellent returns on investment. The industrialisation of healthcare was preceded by the commercialisation of medical education, again starting around 1955. It is in this world that CMCV had to continue in its Ministry of Healing and Education, obeying the command of our Supreme Master. A clear understanding of our heritage, traditions and unique practices is essential as the Institution goes forward in its Ministry in what is becoming an increasingly hostile world.

The inception of the Christian Medical College, Vellore was brought to light on that night, in the last decade of the nineteenth century, in the Mission Bungalow at Tindivanam, a village about 100 km south of Madras (now Chennai), where young Ida was challenged by the desperate need for medically trained women to help the women and children of India. However, the real beginning was an evening in New York in 1818 when Dr. John Scudder, a very successful private practitioner of Medicine, was challenged by the casual reading of a pamphlet titled "The Conversion of the World or the claims of 600,000,000 and the ability and duty of the Churches Respecting them" found in the living room of a patient he was called to see. Dr. John was moved to ask the question 'Why doesn't someone do something about this?' and suddenly a thought flashed in his mind 'Why shouldn't I?' and he heard a voice say 'Go heal the sick and preach the Gospel to those who have never heard of Christ'.

It all started in the 1770s with the life and example of his paternal and maternal grandfathers, one of them a doctor and the other an army colonel. Their influence and the way they responded to the challenges of the American War of Independence held a huge impact. Theirs was the tradition and spirit that guided Dr. John's response to his challenge.

Seven overlapping generations have contributed to the birth, growth and development of CMCV, thus beginning the third decade of the twenty–first century. An eighth and many more generations are waiting in the future. A clear delineation of these generations help to understand better, the evolution of the Christian Medical College, Vellore.

The First Generation: Dr. John Scudder and Mrs. Harriet Waterbury Scudder (1815-1855)

Dr. John Scudder was the first American medical missionary to India. When Dr. John was challenged to commit his life to bring the Gospel to India, it was not an easy decision. His father, a successful businessman in New York, disapproved of his decision and when he persisted further, disinherited him and refused to talk to him. He even refused to read the letters his son wrote from India and threw them in a wastepaper basket! However, it must be mentioned that when his wife retrieved them and read the letters aloud to the other children, the father would sit in the next room with the door open and listen to them! Leaving a lucrative practice and the comforts of New York in 1819, Dr. John, Mrs. Harriet and Maria, their two–year-old daughter boarded the sailing ship *Indus* for a four–month journey around the Cape of Good Hope to India. Their daughter died of dysentery a few days after they landed in Calcutta (now Kolkata). Their next two children also died soon after birth as they struggled to find the way to successfully bring up children in the hostile tropical environment. Mrs. Harriet gave birth to a further ten children, nine of whom survived and came back to work in India as missionaries. Dr. John and Mrs. Harriet worked in Ceylon (now Sri Lanka) and India with only one visit back to the US in 1842, nearly 23 years after they left. The highlight of this visit was reconciliation with Dr. John's father and time with their children who had been sent back for education at the mercy of kindhearted relatives. They returned to India in 1846 where Mrs. Harriet died in 1849 and Dr. John was repatriated for health reasons in 1855 to South Africa, where he died. The challenging and inspiring lives of Dr. John and Mrs. Harriet,certainly, demands a chapter,to be dedicated to them (Appendix 1). Dr. John and Harriet Scudder's response to the challenge to spread the Gospel was the true beginning of CMCV. Christian Medical College Vellore still does not celebrate their seminal role or recognise its real roots as we pass the Bicentenary of his call to India.

The Second Generation: The children who came back (1843-1925)

Apart from Amy, who died soon after their arrival in Calcutta, the John Scudders had twelve more children while in Ceylon and India. The first two of these also died,before they worked out, how to ensure that children survived outside the comforts of New York. Five of the ten survivors had already been sent for education to family members in the USA when they reached the age of around eight to ten years, and the other five returned with their parents in 1842. Nine of the second generation of the Scudders, seven boys and two girls returned to work in India as missionaries. One son died in a swimming accident in the USA while taking theological training to return to India. Five of the seven boys were also qualified medical practitioners, the eldest of them a student of the then newly started Madras Medical College. They along with their wives spent a total of around 400 years of service to India. The last of this generation was Sophia Weld Scudder, the wife of Dr. John Scudder II and the mother of Aunt Ida, who died in Vellore in 1925, after 64 years of service in India. The contributions of this generation included several hospitals, schools, industrial training institutes, etc. (Appendix 2). It is not necessary to detail their work here except that this was the generation into which Ida Sophia Scudder was born in 1870 and who influenced her early life and responses.

The Third Generation: Ida Sophia Scudder and her small group of Pioneers (1850-1918)

December 1870 was a year of double celebration for the John Scudder II family at Ranipet as their only daughter after five sons was born on the 9th. It was a joyous Christmas that year with the parents and the five older brothers doting over Ida Sophia, the new addition to the family. She grew up in India especially through the famine years and the great famine of 1877 in which it is estimated that over 5 million died. The Scudders were responsible for distributing relief supplies and seven–year-old Ida was involved in this, tearing up the limited supply of bread to give the pieces to starving children. The older brothers ensured that the children ate all that they were given and did not smuggle any out to their starving parents outside. The heat, the poverty and dirt of India made a tremendous impression on Ida's young mind and once the family went back for their first furlough in 1877, Ida was determined that she would never come back to this terrible country. 13 years later, as she graduated from school, she was called back to nurse her ailing mother. While she was in Tindivanam, her response to God's challenge through the 'Three Knocks at Night' transformed her life and India. She went back to the USA in 1894, completed her MD and came back to India planning to work with her father, to try and transform the lives of Indian women. Tragically, her father died of cancer a few months after her return and Ida with the help of her mother had to take over his medical work and win the acceptance of the people in Vellore.

The band of devoted helpers, both Indian and foreign who worked with her and her mother from 1900 to establish the Mary Taber Schell Hospital.They helped to develop village outreach work and Compounder (Allied Health Sciences) and Nursing training at Vellore, leading finally to the Missionary Medical School for Women in 1918.They are the pioneers of the Third Generation of CMCV.

The Fourth Generation: The Missionary Medical School for Women (1918-1942)

Starting a medical school to train Indian women for India in a small village was considered by many a foolhardy enterprise in the post–First World War period. In fact, the government authority in Madras, who had to give permission to start the school, told Aunt Ida rather derisively that if she got six students to apply and join they would give her permission. In fact, of the 69 applicants, 18 were selected of whom 14 completed the four– year course, several of them in the top rank of the University. This LMP course was discontinued by the University in 1938. Vellore had by then, trained nearly 250 women licensed medical practitioners, the majority of whom were working in India and the neighbouring countries, many in the government service. Aunt Ida's contributions to India were recognised in the Award of the *Kaiser-i-Hind* gold medal in 1918. The few teachers, mostly missionaries, Indian doctors, nurses and other helpers and the nursing and medical students trained by Aunt Ida are the Fourth Generation of Vellore. None of them are still with us, but their lives are inspiring. The foundation of the life of the College was laid during the 20 years of the Medical School. The School learnt how to overcome insurmountable difficulties in the last four years while struggling to start the MBBS course.

The people who worked shoulder to shoulder with her during this time, her friends and admirers Gertrude Dodd and Dr. Jessie Findlay, were her key associates, who with several others served for shorter terms ensuring that what was envisioned by Ida was transformed to reality.

The Fifth Generation: The Medical College and Coeducation (1942-1960)

Aunt Ida officially 'retired' when she was 76 (in 1946) but as Principal Emeritus she continued to guide the Institution with her prophetic vision and inspirational insights. The transformation of the Missionary Medical School for Women to a coeducational full–fledged Medical College was guided by her. Her firm decision that CMCV was to be a coeducational institution, implemented in 1947, was something she paid a high price for in broken relationships and loss of friends, of whom she felt was betraying the cause of women. Yet, she persisted with her vision.A large faculty were recruited to fulfil university requirements for the College and from 1953, six years after the first ten male students joined, 25 women and 25 men students were admitted each year. The College had an enviable reputation, both for the quality of student training and the excellence of the care offered to patients. In 1942, the year of the 'Quit India' movement, Aunt Ida said prophetically that the future of the Institution depended on it being "Indian owned, Indian administered". Offering medical services that were generally not available in India, to those who could subsidise the treatment of the poor was an added advantage to those who came to Vellore". Stalwarts in their specialised profession joined Vellore,and started new avenues thus, continuing to uphold Aunt Ida's vision of service to all who needed it. Training of undergraduate and postgraduate students were soundly established. Aunt Ida was very much a part of the Campus at College Hill and all students who trained during this period had the privilege of meeting her and being infected by her spirit! The students who were in the College till 1960 belong to the Fifth Generation. Many of them joined the faculty but all had retired by the Centenary year 2000.

The Sixth Generation: The Years of Rapid Growth (1960-2000)

The passing of the inimitable founder of any institution is an epochal event and the death of Aunt Ida on 26 May 1960 was the end of a glorious chapter in the life of this Institution. Nay, it was the beginning of another equally glorious chapter. The forty years between 1960 and 2000, the centenary of Aunt Ida starting her work at Vellore, were years of rapid growth and strengthening of the Institution. It paved the way for the development of several higher speciality services, automation of the laboratory and imaging services,- several firsts in clinical services in India such as neurosurgery, open heart operations, renal dialysis and transplantation, flexible endoscopy, bone marrow transplant, etc. Research was accepted as an essential part of education and endowed chairs were established. Quality assurance practices and standardisation of laboratory tests were initiated for the first time in India at CMCV. There was also a turmoil with the Labour Union activity, attempts by the government to interfere in the Institution and several legal challenges. The leadership with Dr. John Carman at the helm, as Director, in the initial decade were supported by many Indian faculty. They had been directly influenced by Aunt Ida,with the traditions built by her that strengthened the policies and practices which were later codified and established. The student strength was increased to 60 in 1962 and there was rapid growth of the number of different postgraduate programmes, diploma, degree and the so-called higher specialties. From 1970, the administrative leadership was completely Indian. The faculty was clear that what had been imparted to them by the founder and the pioneers who worked with her should be transmitted to the students they were training. All faculty belonging to the Fifth Generation had superannuated by 2000, the Centenary of founding the Hospital. The Institution was in the hands of those who. had no first-hand knowledge of the pioneers and the founder, the Sixth Generation.

The Seventh Generation: Safe Hands for Now and the Future (2000 onwards)

The last Director belonging to the Fifth Generation retired in 1997. The last member of the Fifth Generation on the faculty retired.

Just prior to the Centenary year, the present Director and his four predecessors are from the sixth generation.The faculty and students who joined the Institution after 2000 are the Seventh Generation and they have not had direct contact with the fifth generation who knew the founder. Such transitions are of crucial importance in the life of any institution. It is, therefore, questionable that the Divine Vision given to the founder is challenged. The need of Indian women and children, through the desperate pleas of their husbands and fathers, be preserved and transmitted to people who carry on the work? At an International Consultation in 2016 on the future of the Institution, it was argued vehemently by some members of the sixth generation that the motto of CMCV "Not to be ministered unto, but to minister" should be reviewed and made more contemporary! This suggestion was not accepted by the group and was not part of the recommendations. This episode epitomises the challenges of a changing socio–economic polity. By eflux of time, there will be a generational change when the last of the sixth generation superannuates and we will have the eighth generation, who would have to be motivated and inspired by the seventh. Do we have unique records that will be available for the future generations to use as a guideline ?

Why this Book

"The object of the Association is the establishment and development of a Christian Medical College and Hospitals in India Women and men shall receive an education of the highest grade in the art and science of Medicine and Nursing or even in one or other of the related professions. This is to equip them, in the spirit of Christ for the service and relief of the suffering and in the promotion of sound health."

The above quotation from the 'Memorandum of Association' of The Christian Medical College Vellore Association, registered in 1947 encapsulates the reason for the existence of CMCV. It is a comprehensive guide for the future. Over the last seven decades, action plans, strategies, guidelines, traditions, and rules have been established. Some of them are unique to CMCV. Some are enshrined in the Constitution and By–laws of the Association and other Books of Rules are available to all staff and students. How many, even if they are part of the administrative set up, read and understand the rules? Many are traditions, established by needs and transmitted as the generations change and can be discerned by a variety of resolutions in Council Minutes. Will they be circumvented or broken with impunity?

This book is planned to show how the Institution evolved from a missionary effort with a few Indian partners and is a small beginning to the present, very large complex, spread over six campuses (Schell, Town, Bagayam, KV Kuppam (RUHSA), Kannigapuram and Chittoor). CMCV is owned and administered by the Association, a wholly Indian, registered society with current membership of 53 different Indian Christian churches and Christian organisations. It rests on four Pillars: the students, the patients, the staff and the Association.

Leadership to the large team of doctors, nurses, allied health technologists and other staff is offered by the Director and the team of administrative officers, who carry out the policy guidelines of the Council of the Association. It is an Unaided Minority Educational Institution as defined in Article 30 Section 1 of the Constitution of India. It is self–financing, raising funds following the strategies initiated in 1942 by Aunt Ida. May God guide us to understand His plan and purpose for us, as we trace the growth, development and generational changes in CMCV, India and the World.

Chapter 1

An Evaluation of a Century of Medical Education at CMCV, 2018

Undergraduate medical training was started by Aunt Ida and her colleagues in Vellore in July 1918 when eighteen young girls were selected from 69 applicants. They were accommodated in rented buildings on the Officers Line and laboratory facilities were borrowed from the Voorhees College run by the Arcot Mission. These girls were trained for the licentiate examination (LMP) of the Madras University. Aunt Ida's vision and conviction was that the service she was doing in the Mary Taber Schell Hospital could only be effective if the Hospital was on the basis of not only treating Indian women and children but it be also a vibrant forum to train Indian girls to serve the medical needs of their fellow citizens. How do we evaluate the success of her dream, 100 years later?

The Missionary Medical School for Women began in 1918, with three teachers and 18 students.It has grown into the Christian Medical College Vellore with a medical faculty of over 500, a large nursing and allied health sciences faculty, nearly 1700 doctors, 2700 nurses, 2000 technical staff with appropriate support staff and facilities, spread over six campuses in and around Vellore. The total students enrolled (excluding Distance

Education) were Two Thousand Seven Hundred and Fifty Four (501 for MBBS, 779 in Medical Postgraduate Diploma, Degree and Fellowship Courses, 868 under the Nursing Faculty and 606 in Allied Health Science Degree and Diploma programmes).

From the modest start in a single room on the Mission Compound on the Arni Road, followed by the 40–bed Mary Taber Schell Hospital, the clinical facilities have also expanded exponentially to a total of 2858 in–patient beds, that catered to 25,60,377 out–patients, 1,35,329 in–patients and welcomed 19,668 babies into this world in 2015–2016. The philosophy enunciated by Aunt Ida, provided high quality services for those who can afford to pay to subsidise the care of those who cannot afford.It has guided the Institution to be almost financially self–sufficient. By most standards, the Institution would be considered a great success.The annual evaluations by different publications have ranked CMCV as in the first or second rposition among all medical colleges in India and as the best non–governmental hospital. Is this evaluation justifiable?

Aunt Ida's first trainee in 1900 was Salome Benjamin, the wife of the cook in the Mission Bungalow at Vellore. She trained to be her helper and assistant from the beginning. Salome responded so well to her training that she was appointed as the matron of a ward in the hospital in Thottapalayam when it opened in 1930. Clearly, the first trainee was a success. Has this success continued or adopted?

An evaluation at least 25 years after graduation of the batches of the undergraduates trained at different time periods at Vellore would be one way to measure the success of what Aunt Ida started a century ago. Two classes of students, the last batch who completed their training while Aunt Ida was still an inspiring presence on the campus (The Class of 1955) and a class which was admitted 25 years after her passing away. (The Class of 1985) were asked to evaluate the nature of the undergraduate training at Vellore and the success of Aunt Ida's vision.

The Class of 1955

The third Saturday of June 1955 was a red–letter–day that fifty youngsters (twenty–five women and twenty–five men) can never forget. At an Assembly, in the Sunken Garden on the CMCV Campus at Bagayam, their names were announced as those privileged to spend the next four and a half years training to follow the glorious tradition established by Ida Sophia Scudder. They were privileged to call her Aunt Ida, the visible expression of the motto of the Institution 'Not to be ministered unto, but to Minister'. This was the last class to complete training while Aunt Ida was still an indomitable figure on the campus. Who were these privileged fifty, selected from a hundred– called to Vellore for detailed evaluation after their success in an all–India written examination in which over eight hundred students competed?

They ranged in age from seventeen and a half to just touching thirty. There were 46 Christians including three Catholics, three Hindus and one Parsee. They came from nine different states of India as well as Sri Lanka and Malaysia. In general, they were from modest middle– class families. Very few had doctors in the family and none were the children of the alumni. Many parents were teachers, mission workers or government servants. Very few of them had secured admission in other medical colleges. Almost half, had studied up to school final, in their mother tongue. Four had a Bachelor's degree and one a Master's.

A quarter of the class required scholarships to complete their medical course. They were selected after a rigorous process, evaluating their academic credentials as well as their suitability for training at CMCV. (Appendix 3 describes the process of selection and the undergraduate training in the 1950's.)

So many years had passed since their graduation in 1960,– the year Aunt Ida died. What does their record show? Postgraduate qualifications in a diversity of health sciences were obtained by thirty–eight of the fifty, including four PhDs. Ten became teachers in medical colleges, three giving a lifetime of service to their *alma mater*. Eighteen worked all their life in mission hospitals. Two were elected Fellows of the Indian National Science Academy, the highest national recognition for excellence in research. Twenty–four spent their working years in their country of origin, while the others were dispersed all over the world. Periodic gathering of the class till 2015 showed that wherever they were working, they were still true to the motto of CMCV and rendered service in the spirit of Christ. Graduates of the Class made three unique clinical contributions to India: the first use of the artificial kidney for dialysis (1961), the first renal transplant (1973), and the first flexible gastrointestinal endoscopy (1974).

What was the magic of Vellore that changed these ordinary youngsters to a distinguished group of medical professionals dedicated for service in the spirit of Christ? Their dedication and sincerity of a lifetime of service shows that they can be rest assured that Aunt Ida was proud and grateful for what they had done. They had also handed over the same zeal to their students and colleagues. Their biographies are inspirational, but space permits the summary of only one.

Dr. Stephen Hansdak, MBBS, MS. Class of 1955

One night in early 1880, Palu Hansdak, a Santhal tribal, had to flee his village of Bijaypur in the Santhal Parganas in the then Bengal Presidency of British India. He had to seek refuge with the Norwegian missionaries at Ranga because his villagers were preparing to kill his young wife whom they suspected to be a witch. They were sheltered by the village Pastor in Ranga and eventually became Christians. Palu became the Pastor of Dumaria in due course and worked in that capacity till his death in 1941. Stephen, born in 1931 was the eighth child of Palu's eldest son who worked as a primary school teacher, supplementing his meagre salary in rice farming. His education in a local language school was interrupted after the 3rd year because the family ran out of money and the entire land was in the grip of a famine. The family survived on rice gruel and jackfruits which grew in their yard. A year later, Stephen was sent to the boys' boarding school in Kaerabani run by the Santhal Mission, where he was offered a scholarship. His father paid part of his boarding fees in kind by the produce of his small farm. Stephen was good at his studies and in athletics, becoming the school champion for two consecutive years. Hindi was the medium of instruction and his Principal, Rev. Harold Rieber, an American Missionary saw his potential and encouraged Stephen to join a college in Ranchi with science, including Biology as a subject so that he could try and become a doctor.

It was too late to apply to Vellore for admission in 1954 when he successfully completed the Intermediate course. He went back to his school as a teacher and applied a year later to CMCV. His spoken English was very poor and so he did not do very well at the interview, although his academic record was very good. The evaluation of suitability for training by his group observers during the interview and the strong recommendation from his headmaster and the support of the Church persuaded the College to give him a chance. He justified this confidence and was always one among the top ten students and graduated in 1960 successfully. By that time, he was married to Alice, a Santhal girl who had graduated as a nurse from Ludhiana.

After Stephen completed his internship, the couple joined the Mohulpahari Christian Hospital in the Santhal Parganas, then a part of Bihar. This was a 90–bed hospital started in 1951 as part of the Santhal Mission. The couple worked there till 1965 when Stephen was selected for the postgraduate course in General Surgery at CMCV and was successful, obtaining the MS degree at his first attempt in 1968. Immediately after the success in the examination, the family (now with three children) returned to Mohulpahari and joined the hospital in May 1968. He was made the Medical Superintendent the following year and served the medical and surgical needs of his people. The Santhals,lived in this relatively inaccessible and backward area of India till he finally retired 33 years later at the age of 70. Unfortunately, he died the next year, 2002.

Many years after graduation, Stephen was asked by his classmates for some highlights of his career. During the first week in Mohulpahari, one of his patients a lady in obstructed labour with the second of twins suffered due to a transverse lie. Stephen remembered clearly the instructions of Dr. Jameson, his teacher of Obstetrics, said a prayer and successfully delivered the second twin after an internal podalic version as a breech delivery, a procedure he had never seen done. Mother and babies were fine. One of the more popular operations he was able to do, which was much appreciated, was correction of cleft lips and palate, although he had no training in plastic surgery. He increased the number of beds of the hospital to 130 beds. He started a school of nursing along with his wife and worked with the Christian Medical Association of India. He attended several international conferences of Christian doctors, where his presentations on his work were well accepted and his dedication to his people was commended. All this he accomplished after duty hours for he had to work, on the land they rented as a farm to supplement his meagre income.

Stephen was awarded the Paul Harrison Award for devoted service in needy areas by CMCV in 1988. The last paragraph of the citation sums up his work: *"In recognition of a lifetime of faithful, devoted and effective service in the Spirit of Christ to His own needy people in a remote rural part of our country, the Paul Harrison Award for 1988 is presented to Dr. Stephen Hansdak."*

This remarkable life of a remarkable man epitomises all that Aunt Ida wanted to achieve for India when she started training young Indians to be doctors.

The Class of 1985

A quarter of a century after Aunt Ida's death, the number of students selected each year had increased to 60 including one student nominated by the Ministry of Health, Government of India. Thirty-one young men and twenty-nine young women were selected and admitted in 1985 through a process similar to that for the Class of 55 focussed on assessing suitability for training at Vellore.

They ranged in age from seventeen to twenty–one. There were 51 Christians including two Catholics, seven Hindus, one Muslim, and one Buddhist. They came from fourteen different states of India as well as from Bangladesh and Malaysia. In general, they were from modest middle–class families. Their parents were government servants, teachers, defence personnel, healthcare professionals, or Church workers. Eleven were the children of doctors and three were the children of alumni. They were selected after a rigorous process, evaluating their academic credentials as well as their suitability for training at CMCV, by a process similar to that in 1955.

Evaluating their record in 2015, fifty–three of the sixty had completed postgraduate training and ten were working as faculty in medical colleges, seven in their *Alma Mater*. Thirty–one were still working in their country of origin, the majority in non–metropolitan areas. Twenty–seven were distributed all over the world, including two in Sub–Saharan Africa. All the mission–sponsored students had worked for at least two years in mission hospitals or areas of need. A review by the Class at their 30th year reunion at Vellore in 2015 clearly indicated that the values that they had acquired from their teachers at Vellore were upheld by them in their work. Aunt Ida while inculcating the service to the needy as a primary responsibility of her students, also emphasised that being a Christian doctor meant the pursuit of excellence in their chosen area of work. One such life from the Class of 85 is summarised.

Vikram Mathews

Vikram was the youngest of three children in a middle–class Malayali Christian family. He studied in a Jesuit school in

Bangalore and played for the Karnataka state hockey team before joining Vellore in 1985. CMC offered diverse extracurricular and leadership opportunities, and Vikram graduated with the unusual composite distinction of having been the Best Incoming All–Rounder, Best Outgoing Student in Academics, the Best Athlete, and the President of the Students' Association as well as Mess Secretary of the Men's Hostel.

Vikram then served in a mission hospital in Karnataka and returned to do his post–graduation in Internal Medicine. India's first successful bone marrow transplant programme had been established in Vellore by another 'Best Outgoing' alumnus – Dr. Mammen Chandy of the Batch of 1967. Vellore's generous study and sabbatical leave opportunities enable its junior faculty to obtain training in specialised areas chosen by them at leading international centres of excellence and to bring back their newly acquired skills to their country and *Alma Mater*. Mammen after joining the faculty at Vellore was deputed to train in Haematology in Australia. Returning to the faculty at Vellore, he established an outstanding Department of Haematology and started the first training programme in India leading to the degree of DM in Haematology. In 2001, Vikram became the first Indian–trained Clinical Haematologist. Other alumni of Vellore's DM course lead haematology programmes in academic centres in India and around the world.

The close integration between laboratory and clinical sciences in the Department of Haematology provided the milieu for developing a practice–changing therapy. Arsenic trioxide became a feasible, economical front–line therapy for acute promyelocytic leukaemia. In recognition of over two decades of work on the prognostication, diagnosis and treatment of acute leukemias, Vikram has received the Indian American Association of Cancer's Lifetime Achievement Award for Outstanding Contribution to Haematology; the DBT Wellcome India Alliance Senior Research Award, twice in 2012 and in 2018, and more recently its prestigious Team Science Grant. He also is the lead investigator of the ICMR designated 'Center of Advanced Research' in acute myeloid leukaemia. He has been elected Fellow of the Indian Academy of Science. As a busy Clinical Haematologist, a researcher investigating mechanisms of drug resistance in leukaemia, with over 200 publications, Vikram is the current Director of the Christian Medical College, Vellore. Almost 40 years after joining CMC, Vikram continues to excel in diverse domains.

Is CMCV fulfilling the objectives of the founder

The Memorandum of Association of the Institution, registered in 1947 when Aunt Ida was a member of the Governing Council, clearly states the objective of the Institution to be a place "… where women and men may receive an education of the highest grade in the Art and Science of Medicine and of Nursing, to equip them, in the spirit of Christ, for service in the relief of suffering and the promotion of health. "

When Aunt Ida recognised the potential of Salome Benjamin and trained her as her assistant, she was only following the tradition that had been begun by her grandfather and her uncles who had trained several young men to be their assistants. A more systematic training was started by her when Mrs. Gnanambal, a trained Pharmacist joined her after the Hospital opened. This was followed by the nurses training programme beginning in

1909. Clearly, the objective was to maximise the impact of the Healing Ministry of Christ by increasing the available human resources. From the first batch of medical students in 1918, the selection criteria was the suitability for training in the Spirit of Christ for the service in the relief of suffering and the promotion of health. By the time recruitment to the Diploma programme in the Missionary Medical School for Women had to be stopped in 1938, because of a policy decision by the government to abolish that programme and train only for the MBBS Degree, over 250 young women had been selected, trained, motivated and sent out to carry the message of Vellore throughout India and in other lands. This was much appreciated and was the basis of the *Kaiser-e-Hind* award to Aunt Ida.

The analysis given above clearly shows that the system of selection by assessing suitability for training at Vellore in the light of the objectives of the Institution and the almost Gurukulam–like fully residential training for the MBBS programme has taken average students and turned them into motivated individuals, who have taken the motto of CMCV to the world. Many graduates from Vellore become teachers inspired by the vision of Aunt Ida that if you train people in the Healing Ministry, you maximise the impact. The high proportion of teachers in both the batches of graduates described here indicates that transmission of the mission to train that was Aunt Ida's, is still a major motivating factor at Vellore in addition to excellence of care. Clearly, the Spirit of Aunt Ida is still the driving force at the Christian Medical College Vellore.

Chapter 2

The Seed is Sown

December 9, 1870 was a day of rejoicing for the family of Dr. John Scudder II when their only daughter, Ida Sophia Scudder was born. Dr. John, his wife Sophia Weald Scudder and their five sons were at Ranipet near Vellore, where he was in charge of the Arcot Mission Hospital. The Scudder family, starting in 1819 with Dr. John Scudder Sr. and his wife Harriet, who by then had completed over 50 years of service in India. All their nine surviving children had served or were serving in India. They had founded The American Arcot Mission of the Reformed Church in America. They established schools and industrial training institutes and did medical work. A hospital was established in Ranipet by Dr. John Scudder II in an old British Army barracks. In 1870, twelve members of the Scudder family were serving the Arcot Mission.

Ida grew and thrived. She was a source of great joy to the family. Her brothers teased their younger sister and she competed with them and was not behind them in any childhood mischief.

Dr. John Scudder II and family moved to Vellore and occupied the large Mission Bungalow on the outskirts of town. He practised medicine and preached the Gospel. He visited the homes of patients or in the village churches that the Arcot Mission had founded. Preaching the Gospel and administering the Arcot Mission took more time than his medical work. All this work was overwhelmed by the great famine of 1877–78. John was tasked with supervising the distribution of relief material by the government and had to tour the entire district. Mrs. Sophia had to supervise the work in town and recruited her children to help in feeding the local children in a camp on the Mission Compound. Their job was to distribute the small amounts of the bread, biscuits and porridge to emaciated, starving children while their parents were kept outside the Compound. They had to ensure that the children ate all that they were given and did not smuggle out any food to their parents. The dust, dirt, heat and deaths during this period made an indelible impression about the undesirability of working in India on little Ida's mind. It was with relief that she went on furlough to America with her family in 1878.

The family spent four happy years at their farm in Nebraska, while Dr. John slowly recovered from the ravages of hard work without any rest in the tropical environment. It was a happy time of family bonding and growing up. The eldest son was sent to a boarding school, while the younger five including Ida attended the nearest village school 8 km away, travelling back and forth on the single horse they possessed. In 1882, Dr. John went back to continue work at the Arcot Mission. Mrs. Sophia stayed back to look after the children but was sorely missed by Dr. John. Two years later, in 1884 she decided to join her husband and the children, as was the practice in the Scudder family,who at that time lived with their aunts and uncles. Fourteen–year–old Ida was to stay with her eldest uncle Rev. Dr. Henry Martin Scudder. Although well looked–after, she had a sense of abandonment and despair when her mother left for India. This reinforced her determination to have nothing to do with India when she grew up. Within a year, Uncle Henry decided to go as a missionary to Japan and the question was what to do with Ida. At the suggestion of Rev. Dr. DL Moody, she was admitted to the Northfield Academy founded by him at his birthplace in Massachusetts.

The years at the Northfield Academy were happy years spent in making new friends, getting a liberal education and being game for any mischief that came her way! In fact, the experience of being disciplined at Northfield helped her when she was responsible to look after the high spirited girls in the Missionary Medical School for Women. Even after she had officially retired, her tolerance for mischief by students was shown in the way she responded. When confronted one day, at breakfast she was sharing with the then Principal and her niece Dr. Ida Belle Scudder, by the MBBS Class of 1955 who were in the process of happily breaking many rules. Her first response before the Principal could launch into a disciplinary harangue, was "Let us kneel and pray that these children would be safe". This prayer saved the students from serious disciplinary action! Life at Northfield strengthened her determination that she would not be just another Scudder Missionary to India. Ida was beautiful, high spirited, athletic and good at her studies as well as deeply Christian. She had many friends from Northfield and many admirers from the companion Boys Academy at nearby Mount Hermon. Ida graduated from Northfield in 1880 fully determined to make a life for herself in America.

The Call and the Response

A telegr from her father in India calling her to come and nurse her ailing mother changed all her plans. She joined the Arcot Mission as a short service missionary and sailed for India along with her brother Harry who had decided to work in the Arcot Mission. Landing in Madras and meeting her father after eight long years was a great joy. The trip by train to Tindivanam and the dusty bullock cart ride from the station to the house reinforced her conviction that this was not the country for her. The sight of starving children brought back the memories of the great famine, strengthening her determination to return to America as soon as her mother recovered. The joyful welcoming embrace of her mother washed away all the hurt and loss of the six years that they had been separated and Ida again became the daughter of the family.

She quickly got into the routine, taking over many responsibilities from her mother. She enjoyed teaching in the girls school, playing the little organ at services and had taken over much of her mother's work in the house and for the residents of the school. Missionary journeys that she undertook with her father exposed her to the countryside and showed her the evangelistic side of the work of the Mission. One particular journey to Thiruvannamalai to preach during the annual Karthigai Deepam festival along with her uncle Jared and his daughter Dixie was particularly traumatic as it exposed her to the religious hostility of the predominantly Hindu crowd. Experiences like this reinforced her determination not to end up as just another Scudder Missionary in India.

Three young men who dared to break tradition because of their love and concern for their young wives challenged Ida and her response changed the course of History. It is best described in Ida's own words:

"As I sat alone at my desk, in my room in the little bungalow, I heard steps coming up to the verandah and looking up, I saw a very tall and fine-looking Brahmin gentleman. I asked him what I could do for him, and he said his little wife, a mere child, was in labour and having a very difficult time and the untrained barber's wife had said that they could do nothing for her, and asked if I would go and help her. I told him that I knew absolutely nothing about midwifery cases but that my father was a doctor and that when he returned from a call he would gladly come and help. The man drew himself up and said, 'Your father come into my caste home and take care of my wife! She had better die than have anything like that happen.'

Later, I took him over to my father's study and together we pleaded with him. I told him that I would do everything in my power to help his wife, with my father, if he would only let us come! I would be an assistant! Still, he refused. Father also urged him, but he went away, apparently very unhappy because I could not help.

I went to my desk very much stirred by that first encounter. After a time, I heard steps again on the verandah and jumped up, hoping that the man had returned to take my father and me, but instead of seeing the Brahmin gentleman, I saw a Mohammedan who had come to see me, and I was horrified to hear the same plea from him. His wife was dying, a mere child, and would I come and help? Again I said I knew nothing about midwifery cases. I took him to my father, and we both reasoned with him and I said that I would go with my father who was a doctor, and do what I could do to help. A scornful answer made my heart sad. He utterly refused, saying that no man outside his family had ever looked upon the face of his wife.

'She had better die than have a man come into the house,' he said. Again my father and I urged him to allow us to come, but again he refused repeating that she had better die than have a strange man look upon her face; and he left.

I went back to my room with my heart so burdened that I hardly knew how to overcome it. After some time of thinking and trying to get my mind back onto my book, I again heard footsteps, and running to the door, looked out to see if the second man had come back, but again I was more than horrified to have the same plea coming from a third man, a high-caste Hindu. He refused just as the others had done and vanished in the darkness.

I could not sleep that night – it was too terrible. Within the very touch of my hand were three young girls dying because there was no woman to help them. I spent much of the night in anguish and prayer. I did not want to spend my life in India. My friends were begging me to return to the joyous opportunities of a young girl in America, and I somehow felt I could not give that up. I went to bed only in the early morning hours after praying much for guidance. I think that was the first time I ever met God face to face, and all that time it seemed He was calling me into this work.

Early in the morning I heard the 'tom–tom' beating in the village and it struck terror in my heart, for it was a death message. I sent our servant who had come up early, to the village to find out the fate of these three women, and he came back saying that *all of them had died during the night. As a funeral procession passed our house in the the morning, it made me very unhappy.*

I could not bear to think of these young girls as dead.

Again, I shut myself in my room and thought very seriously about the condition of the Indian women. After much thought and prayer, I went to my father and mother and told them that I must go home and study Medicine, and come back to India to help such women."

Death during childbirth was common in the nineteenth century India. It was only during the latter half of the twentieth century, after Independence, that maternal death rates started to come down. God used these three men as His instruments to challenge and call Ida for His purposes. They had to overcome three culturally ingrained hurdles to call for help and it must have been the deep love they had for their wives that gave them the courage. The first was the fear of what the unknown foreigner would do. Having seen the medical work of Dr. John would have helped them to get over this hurdle. The second was the fear that by the touch of the foreigner they would be polluted. The Brahmin and the high–caste Hindu would have known that if their wives survived, there were rituals (*poojas*) that was essential to cleanse her from the pollution. The real barrier was the patriarchal nature of the Indian social structure that saw the wife as the exclusive property of the husband – No other man should see her as she is 'my exclusive possession'. The three men were educated and could converse with Ida in English. They could accept that western medicine may help where indigenous practices failed. Religious and caste taboos could be overcome but they were unable to overcome their cultural patriarchal prejudices. It is unfortunate that even today much of the problems that affect Indian society arise from this patriarchal frame of mind. Even though by the middle of the twentieth century many of the leading practitioners of Obstetrics in India were men There are still many who insist on women doctors to tend their wives.

Ida was confronted by God and chose the better portion and He abundantly blessed her. Although her parents were happy at her decision, she could not rush back to America to start her medical training. She had to wait for the full recovery of her ailing mother and the scheduled home furlough in 1894 to start on the real mission of her life, All this ensured that she was not "just another Scudder Missionary in India". She did assist her father in his medical work at times and spent time at the Arcot Mission Hospital in Ranipet which her father had started in abandoned barracks. She assisted her cousin Dr. Lew Scudder who assured her that she could certainly become a doctor for she was able to complete the sewing up after a major surgery.

Becoming a Doctor

Ida enrolled in the Women's Medical College in Philadelphia in 1895 after passing the Regents examination in New York. Her training in Northfield in liberal arts had ill–prepared her for the science of medicine but with a group of her classmates she embarked on the course enthusiastically. The Women's Medical College was fully accredited offering the MD degree after a four– year course. However, they had a problem. They did not have an affiliated general hospital and their students had to go to general hospitals affiliated to other colleges in Philadelphia to complete their training. The decision by Cornell in 1898 to open their doors to women medical students found Ida and a few others deciding to change over to Cornell for better clinical training in their final year. Although there were initial fears about their reception by the men students, they were welcomed and graduated a year later.

There was an interlude, when the reality of being a woman intruded into Ida's single-minded pursuit of becoming a good doctor to help the women of India. Burchfield Milliken, a young man,training to become a doctor in the Philadelphia Medical College and Ida became good friends. He was concerned when she decided to move to New York as they would be separated. The friendship continued during the busy year at Cornell. After they both graduated, he proposed to Ida, but he was not prepared to be a missionary in India. Ida was not prepared to give up her call to serve the women of India and she was not sure she loved Burchfield Milliken enough to spend the rest of her life with him. They decided to continue as friends. Milliken remained faithful to her, corresponded regularly with her as her dear friend and died of tuberculosis in 1904 while Ida was in India.

Preparing for India

Ida's priorities were clear. She was to join her father at Vellore as soon as possible. Instead of doing a year of internship in New York to refine her clinical skills, she would learn from her father whose knowledge of medicine in the tropics was deeper than that of any of the New York doctors. A fresh challenge came at this time as Dr. Louisa Hart, a graduate of the Women's Medical College, already working at Ranipet convinced the Mission Board that Ida should raise enough funds to build a hospital for women and children at Vellore. Ida suggested that she raise 50,000 dollars for the hospital, but the more realistic Board authorised her to raise up to $8000 for this purpose.

Ida drew up plans enthusiastically with the Women's Auxiliary of the Board and soon realised that while all listened to her with interest, very few actual dollars materialised and the time for her to leave for India was rapidly drawing near. The two elderly ladies with whom she was staying in New York suggested that she make a presentation to the Missionary Society of the Collegiate Church which they attended and present a preliminary talk to Miss Taber who was the President and who lived nearby. Ida walked over and was welcomed by Miss Taber who introduced her to her brother–in–law Mr. Schell and talked to her in the next room. After listening to Ida she invited her to the meeting and was cautiously optimistic that there would be some support.

The next morning at breakfast, she got a note from Mr. Schell asking whether she would meet him before she went to meet the Church group. Ida went over to the house with trepidation and hope that he would give a contribution, maybe as much as a thousand dollars. Mr. Schell asked her many probing questions on the practical aspects of what she hoped to do and about Vellore and the challenges and opportunities there. Finally, he asked what an inexperienced student just out of medical school would be able to achieve. Ida answered that it would be at least a year before the hospital could be built and that she was going to work with her father who had more than two decades of experience of being a doctor in India and that she would learn more about what was relevant to India with him, than in a year's internship in New York. She asked him to check with Cornell about her academic credentials. Suddenly, Mr. Schell smiled and said, "I have already done so' and opened his cheque book and wrote saying, "I have decided to make a contribution to your hospital in memory of my beloved wife, Mary Taber Schell. She would have understood and liked this thing you are trying to do. You're asking, I understand for eight thousand. I want it to be a good hospital, worthy of the memory of a good woman." He pushed the cheque across to her and Ida was stunned speechless when she saw that it was for ten thousand dollars!

The next day, Mr. Schell took Ida downtown to the medical equipment shops and bought all the equipment and fittings that would make the hospital complete. He ordered that it be packed and ready for shipment by the same ship Ida was sailing on. When God gives, He gives abundantly.

At the meeting at the Centennial Church, there was great rejoicing and Ida pleaded that they support an evangelist too for the hospital. Her classmate Annie Hancock, who graduated with her from Northfield, was keen to go out with Ida and work with the women in the hospital and in their homes. She spoke of the urgent need for such work and of her friend who had a calling to this work. At the end of her talk, many of the women came to her with questions and offerered support but it was clear that this was for the future. When all had left, a small woman in dark clothes whose eyes had been a source of encouragement for Ida while she was talking, came up to her and introduced herself as Miss Gertrude Dodd and said that she and her two sisters had decided to support Annie to go out with Ida. Ida hugged her and said that she didn't know how to thank her. Miss Dodd replied that she already had. This was the beginning of a friendship that went on for many decades and made a great difference in the growth and development of the Ministry at Vellore.

Ida was now ready to sail to India on the 22nd of November 1899, the beginning of her life's work and to bring a great transformation in India.

Chapter 3

Train Indian Girls to Look after their Sisters and Children

"You are not building a Medical College.
You are building the Kingdom of God."

– Ida S Scudder

Personal tragedy welcomes Ida to India

Ida and Annie arrived in Vellore on New Year 1900. It was wonderful to be with her parents again and she was impatient to start working with her father. Unfortunately,there were two problems. The first was that patients were not willing to accept her ministrations in the clinic but insisted that they would wait for her father. The prejudice against a woman doctor was not confined to America but was equally or more prevalent in India. Ida was able to go to a few houses to see sick women. The first such call was to see the moribund mother of a rich high– caste Hindu. While her ministrations made the old lady more comfortable before her death, the news of her failure to cure spread fast. The second home visit several days later was more successful, but it was overtaken by the second problem, the rapidly failing health of her father.

The increasing heat as the year progressed to February and March, worsened the health of Dr. John Scudder and the family decided to go to Kodaikanal, a hill station in the Palani Hills near Madurai, earlier than usual. Going up the hills carried in chairs by local labourers or on ponies was an enjoyable experience as it allowed them to escape from the enervating heat of the plains. There was some perceptible improvement in her father's health during the first few days of stay there. He continued to do his work as the Treasurer of the Arcot Along with the mission there Ida revelled in a spate of activities and sports. By May, Dr. John's condition deteriorated and the doctors, including his nephew Dr. Lew Scudder of Ranipet, who was there on holiday, decided that the only chance was an immediate operation. There are no records of the diagnosis or details of the operation. A makeshift operation theatre was set up in the house where they were staying; unfortunately, the doctors found that it was inoperable and Dr. John Scudder II moved on to be with his Maker, the day after the surgery. The eulogies at his funeral, paid tributes to his contributions as a missionary and doctor. It left Ida stunned with the realisation that she now had nobody to introduce her to her life work of caring for Indian women.

A modest beginning

Ida and her mother Mrs. John returned to the Mission Bungalow in Vellore. Ida set up a clinic on the ground floor in a small room with a window where she could dispense medicines. Initially, there were no patients but gradually a trickle started and by the end of summer she was running a busy out–patient treatment programme. She discovered that Salomi Benjamin, the wife of her cook who helped in the kitchen, was an able and quick learner and keen to assist her. Salomi was Ida's first student and quickly became an able helper and essential support for her clinical work. A typical workday started with house visits to the rich and high–caste houses to see women who were reluctant to come to the clinic. She opened the clinic at 8.00 in the morning. She would see and treat around 100 patients with Salomi's help before she had her breakfast around noon. Minor surgery such as lancing abscesses, amputation of infected and gangrenous fingers and small superficial growths were done followed by more house visits in the afternoon. Sore eyes, earache, decayed teeth, skin diseases and fevers were common. Very sick women would be admitted in a small room next to the clinic which should have had only one bed, but necessity made her cramp in three. Malaria and tuberculosis were common serious problems. While quinine could cure the former, the majority of tuberculosis patients came very late and inexorably progressed to death in those days, long before anti-tuberculous treatments were available. Her most difficult task was to explain to the patient and relatives that nothing could be done when inevitably, patients were brought too late. One of her triumphs was when she was called to a house where a girl was dying in childbirth and her ministrations were able to save her and the baby boy. She began to feel that she was partially compensating for the lives lost that night ten years earlier when she was challenged to respond to the needs of the women in India.

The plans for the Mary Taber Schell Hospital were completed and the foundation stone was laid on September 7, 1901 and work started on building the first Women and Children's Hospital in Vellore. Along with the additional responsibility of supervising the construction, she was confronted with a famine and its effect since the monsoons failed completely that year in southern India. The effect of starvation on an already malnourished population compounded the severity of all diseases and Ida was forced to find additional room for her patients. In addition to the essential correspondence with the Mission Board in New York and close family and friends, there was a desultory correspondence with Burchfield Millikken, who developed pulmonary tuberculosis in early 1902. She continued the correspondence with him as a friend till he died of his illness in 1904 leaving her wondering whether he ever meant anything more than a friend.

Mary Taber Schell Hospital

The Mary Taber Schell Hospital building was completed along with a spacious house for her mother and herself and inaugurated the same on 16 September 1902. In two years, she opened a small dispensary,. at the Mission Compound on Arni Road in Vellore She had treated over 5000 patients and made hundreds of house visits and had earned a reputation as a doctor for women. Women from villages, miles away, came for help and none were disappointed with her care, although many were past the point where she could offer anything other than some symptomatic relief along with her loving kindness. She had to run the Hospital initially with only Salomi to help her, as Dr. Louisa Hart who had initiated the idea of Ida starting a women's hospital at Vellore could not join her. Her ill health forced her to go on furlough to America. Soon Mrs. Gnanambal, a trained compounder joined and was in charge of the dispensing all medications. A trained Indian nurse, Mrs. Gnanasundaram, was working along with Salomi in the wards and the clinic.

Her first major challenge was a woman who needed a lifesaving hysterectomy, an operation she had never done alone. She was worried because she had never done any major surgery without a senior colleague to guide her. Her mother placed the problem in perspective by reminding her that if she did not do the operation, the patient would die. Ida did her first major surgery in Vellore assisted by Salomi with the help from the local government hospital to give chloroform for anaesthesia. The successful operation was the first of many with the work in the Hospital, steadily increasing. Dr. Louisa Hart returned from her medical furlough bringing her sister Lilian, a trained nurse. Although, both of them were assigned to Vellore, there was enough work for five doctors. The news of the availability of women doctors had spread widely and women were coming from villages as far away as 50 miles, more than a day's journey away in those days when transportation was primitive. In 1906, they did nearly 300 operations with 800 in- patients and 30,000 patients visiting and getting treatment at the clinic.

The beginning of training – Compounders and Nurses

Salomi, was the first who was trained by her to assist her with all patients including the first major operation,and training a team was one of Ida's priorities. Mrs. Gnanambal, who was her trusted co–worker was in charge of all medication given at the Hospital. She started training compounders to assist her in 1903 and in a year she had reliable people to help her. Ida, Salomi and Mrs. Gnanasundaram selected a few girls and trained them to help in the Hospital to look after the patients. Training uneducated girls from Vellore and nearby villages to follow the exacting standards expected by Ida was a difficult job and the turnover was high. Lilian Hart tried to formalise the training of nurses further, especially as they found that hiring so called trained nurses from other hospitals was worse than their experiences with their own girls.

Ida was increasingly becoming aware of the impact of local customs and traditions on the health of women in India. She found that families advised by her were willing to try and follow her instructions, but ingrained religious and cultural practices came in the way. Established practices like child marriage and the Temple Devadasi system and more directly the patriarchal mindset which saw women as mere chattels of the men were forces that Ida, despite her enthusiasm, was ill equipped to deal with. Her experiences convinced Ida that it was essential to train Indian women to look after their sisters. As she was approaching her furlough back to America in 1907, the thought crystallised in her mind that she must start a school of nursing to train young women to go out to live with the people and show them better ways of living. She also planned an initiative to take medicine to the villages around Vellore and realised she would need a car to do this roadside ministry more effectively. A school of nursing was a major new venture requiring teachers, new buildings and acceptance. All of this would need a lot of money, but an equally important question was, who would come to be trained as nurses?

Ida left on furlough with her mother and Annie in November 1907. The Harts and the devoted Indian team of Salomi, Mrs. Gnanambal and Sr. Gnanasundaram kept the work going at Vellore. They and the patients felt Ida's absence acutely. The furlough was no holiday, travelling the breadth of America and Canada, speaking to groups to raise funds for her work and especially for a school of nursing and a car to take medicine out to villages. Funds were raised and a small car for village work was ordered to be shipped to Vellore. Ms. Delia Houghton, a registered nurse, was recruited by the Mission to look after the Hospital and to start a school of nursing.

Ida was particularly delighted to renew her friendship in person with Miss Gertrude Dodd, who had funded Annie Hancock's travel to Vellore and kept up regular correspondence with Ida. Ida stayed with her while in New York and suggested to Miss Dodd that she should visit Vellore and learn the work at first hand, as she was the Treasurer of her Mission Board. She needed little persuasion to agree and along with her friend Katherine van Nest, with whom Ida used to stay when she studied at Cornell, booked tickets to go to Vellore. The only break during this period was a holiday with the family on the Nebraska farm where she had enjoyed several years as a child. Miss Dodd tried to make up for this with a leisurely trip through Europe where she could show her friend the Europe she loved. While enjoying Europe, Ida was anxious to get back to Vellore where her world waited for her.

Waiting for the new car to arrive, Ida started her village outreach programme, going to Gudiyattam and to distant Punganoor about 80 miles away where her brother Harry had a Mission station. She could do this because Louisa Hart was there. Such a journey by train and horse cart (Jutka) meant she was away at least four night.Dr. Louisa Hart left on furlough in March 1909. The presence of her friend Gertrude Dodd was a great source of strength for her. It also offered her companionship more than what her mother gave. Miss Dodd also shouldered much of Ida's administrative responsibilities as she had a flair for business.

She left for America in September 1909, soon after the School of Nursing was opened.The first class were with five new girls along with the girls who were already trained by Ida. Delia Houghton was an excellent teacher, who maintained high standards.

The Germ of the Idea

The car – a Peugeot – arrived, was uncrated and assembled and the routine of weekly trips to Gudiyattam with stops on the way out and way in where patients would assemble for treatment, was gradually established. This was the beginning of the roadside clinics of Vellore. Other villages were visited periodically and the need for increasing the roadside work was clear but there was only so much Ida could do. The work at the Mary Taber Schell Hospital increased in volume and complexity. It appeared that Ida Scudder's mission to help the women of India had taken off, but there was a nagging discomfort in her mind. The more she achieved, the more she realised the enormity of the task and the limitation of what one woman with a few dedicated locally trained girls could accomplish. At that time, while there was one doctor for every 600 people in America, in India it was less than one per 10,000. The first Tamil woman to become a doctor, Muthulaxmi Reddy, had just graduated from the Madras Medical College in 1909.

The facilities at the Mary Taber Schell Hospital were becoming inadequate for the work.So Ida requested the Board for $3000 for additions to the buildings. While she was writing the letter, it struck her that it was not extensions to the hospital she needed but a medical college to train Indian women to be doctors. At the 1911 annual summer Missionary Medical Conference at Kodaikanal, where most of the missionary doctors working in southern India from different denominational missions attendent, Ida boldly proposed that they formally approve the founding of a Union Medical College for Women and requested that they start making plans for it immediately. Many in the group were sceptical but she was supported by Dr. Anna Kugler, who had established a hospital for women at Guntur for the Lutheran Church and Dr. McPhail of the Free Church of Scotland. There were objections, mainly from men,which ranged from the possibility of not getting any women to train to the enormous cost of such an endeavour with the missions always struggling for money, Drs Scudder, Kugler and McPhail managed to persuade the group to appoint a committee to study and bring back recommendations next year.

When they met again in 1912, Ida was not there as she could not get cover for the work at Vellore while she went to Kodaikanal. The Committee had done their work well and all at the conference agreed that there should be a Union Medical College for Women in southern India. The idea was accepted although most of the male doctors felt it would never be achieved, all that remained was to choose a place, get permission and some financial support from the Colonial Government and persuade the parent missions that this was a priority for which funds must be raised. Ida was thrilled with this decision. She already had identified a site about 4 miles south of Vellore town where there were about 200 acres of barren land on which she could see the medical college thriving. Meanwhile, how could she raise almost a million dollars that would be needed to ensure that Vellore could begin this endeavour?

Her health failed in mid–1913 and she was advised to take a holiday in Kodaikanal. She was forced to rest and contemplate as advised by Burchfield Milliken in his last letter:*"Take time from your little detailed work to contemplate the vast worldwide centuries in/of long things"*. The words of her favourite hymn became the motivating and driving force of her life in a very real way.

"Be Thou my vision, O Lord of my heart." Naught be all else to me, save that Thou art. Thou my best thought, by day or by night; Waking or sleeping, Thy presence my light."

Ida came back from this period of rest with renewed energy not only for her work at the Hospital but also to plan for the college.

New friends, new possibilities

It was at this point that God opened a new door. Lucy Peabody, the only woman representative from America at the International Missionary Council in Holland that year, was commissioned to investigate the suitability of Madras as the site for a Union Christian Arts College for women,.It was one among half a dozen women's colleges that the Council hoped to support in Asia. Lucy Peabody and her companions spent 24 hours on an unscheduled visit to Ida Scudder in Vellore, and by the end of the day had caught Ida's vision of training Indian women to be doctors and committed to work with her to raise funds. Ida was no longer alone in her drive to start the Medical School for Women at Vellore but had found a dynamic ally for fundraising.

Lucy Peabody even visited and enthusiastically approved the proposed site of the college at Bagayam about four miles south of Vellore Town.

Ida was working with renewed energy towards her vision of a medical college for women. She needed at least a 150–bed hospital to support the college. The patients at the Mary Taber Schell Hospital was steadily increasing and she realised that there was no land there to build a larger hospital. Her persistence paid off and finally the Board in New York gave permission for her to raise money during her furlough in 1914. Her persistence also persuaded the Colonial Government in Madras to sanction a grant of $20,000 if she raised matching funds of $40,000. She had powerful allies in Lucy Peabody, Katherine van Nest in America and the Principal of the Mission's Voorhees College in Vellore. It was the Board's approval of buying new land for the hospital in the centre of the town about a mile and a half from the Schell facility in March 1914. She took it as a positive sign, but of course they did not sanction enough money. They advised that she could apply for the government grant and that she be patient and wait till her furlough to raise money for the college!

There were other good news too The South India Missionary Association recommended that a Union Medical School for Women be established at Vellore in connection with the Hospital.They wished that Ida Scudder be the Principal and that she represents the Committee in a fundraising campaign in the United States and in Britain. Ida sailed on furlough in July 1914, leaving Dr. Lilian Cook in charge of the Hospital with her trusted Indian colleagues. Before she disembarked in New York, the First World War had broken out and with Europe in flames, the fundraising issue had changed. With a whole year of campaigning in US and Canada,all she and Lucy Peabody could raise was $10,000. She also got the gift of a Ford car to continue the roadside clinics and her outreach programme to take medicines to the needy villages. The Peugeot was almost worn out and had become very unreliable. The happiest outcome of this furlough wait was that Gertrude Dodd, her closest friend and Treasurer of the Mission Board, decided that her commitment to the Mission work of her Church would be best fulfilled if she moved permanently to Vellore to help Ida in her work. The other,was the resolute Lucy Peabody, continued the campaign for the seven women's colleges in South and East Asia, among which the Women's Medical College at Vellore was included.

The Medical School

Ida came back to Vellore via the Pacific in 1915 and plunged into her busy medical work. This was increased by the threats of a raging plague epidemic and the debates that continued in New York with the Board and in southern India at the Interdenominational Missionary Medical Association on whether the College should be interdenominational and whether women could make the grade in medical education. In the meantime, plans for the buildings were being prepared. The government approved in principle, to the starting of the School and the Board approved of Ida paying for an option on the land in Bagayam where she planned to build the College and Hospital. More land was purchased in the centre of the town next to the Jutka stand where a clinic and in future more wards could be built.

The War in Europe had its impact in India with rising costs, scarce supplies, and the involvement of the Indian Army in the War. Ida found that the work load in the Mary Taber Schell Hospital steadily increased as her fame as a doctor spread, and with the new car, she increased the outreach work. Even with other doctors to help her, she often spent 24–hour work days. However, despite her preoccupation with increased work and the clinical challenges, her thoughts were constantly on how the College could become a reality. She did not believe in waiting for things to happen but knew that the best way to start was to begin the same, by herself. All the permissions for the College, including from the Board in New York, were with her. What was lacking was the money and the go–ahead signal from the Presidency Medical Department. Early in 1918, while the War still raged in Europe, Ida met Colonel Bryson, the S urgeon General, Head of the Medical Department of Madras Presidency, to discuss the possibility of starting a medical school to give the LMP diploma after four years of training. She had plans to rent buildings for a hostel and classrooms and had arranged for the Voorhees College to give classes in Chemistry and Physics, an essential part of the first –year curriculum.

Although, he started as a sceptic,after the persuasive presentation by Ida, Col. Bryson gave formal permission for her to start the course with, at least six applicants which could go upto twenty five candidates.

The prospectus she drafted and dispatched showed that while she was calling for applicants for the LMP course, the plan was to start a full–fledged MBBS programme,once the War was over and the necessary infrastructure was in place. She started an active recruitment drive and got a total of sixty–nine applicants, from whom only eighteen met the high standards set by Ida. Four of them dropped out due to various reasons and when the School was opened on August 12, 1918 by the Governor of the Madras Presidency, Lord Pentland, there were only fourteen. The words of Colonel Bryson at the inaugural function were prophetic: *"I wonder if you realize what important people you are. Fifty years hence, you will remind the students of that generation that you were among those present at the opening of this school. It is an honour that none can ever share with you."*

Indeed, in August 1968 Aunt Ida and none of her first batch of students were present at Vellore on the Golden Jubilee of the start of medical education. It was recognised that it was an honour to be a student at the Christian Medical College Vellore, which by then was admitting 60 undergraduate students each year and had over 60 students in postgraduate training programmes and an enviable reputation as a medical centre where the finest of clinical care was provided ethically without consideration of caste or creed.

Conclusion

There were many hands involved in the pursuit of health professional training for women in India. Ida was the driving force with her determination that Indian women should be trained to look after their sisters and children. The support of her mother, who after the tragic loss of her husband came back to the Mission Bungalow in Vellore and supported Ida to carry on the work of her father. This was the key element that freed Ida from the mundane chores of the household and enabled her to pursue her God given dream. Her mother gave Ida the strength and courage to pioneer, in the same way that she guided her to do the first hysterectomy at the Mary Taber Schell Hospital. The host of Indians who worked with Ida starting with Salomi, Mrs. Gnanambal, Sister Gnanasundaram and Hussain, the driver and others whose names we do not know, were essential partners in pursuing Ida's Vision. The story of Thungammah who worked in the Hospital for five rupees a month as a sweeper,and over the years saved 69 rupees from her meagre salary. This, she triumphantly gave it to Ida for purchasing a pump for the new hospita,Certainly, the sacrificial act epitomises the commitment and faithfulness of the Indian partners. Starting with Annie Hancock, Louisa and Lilian Hart and others who worked with Ida at the Mary Taber Schell Hospital and Lucy Peabody who raised the funds, there were many missionaries who helped to fulfil Ida's dream. The role of Ms. Gertrude M. Dodd, after whom the Dodd Memorial Library in the Town Campus at Vellore is name, was that she devoted her life and a considerable fortune to be with Ida to help her fulfil her vision, was invaluable, but probably not given due recognition.

In 1878, eight–year–old Ida going on furlough to the United States of America felt that she was escaping from a country of dirt, poverty and misery to which shewould nevercomeback. She came back 12 years later to nurse her mother. God challenged her with the reality of life of women in India and Ida responded to the challenge, trained to become a doctor and came back to India at the beginning of the 20th Century to address the health needs of women. She quickly realised the need to train Indian women to be health professionals and after starting schools of pharmacy (to train compounders) and nursing she was obsessed with starting a medical college for women. She was a pioneer in interdenominational co-operation and managed to inspire the different denominational missionaries in Southern India.

She also initiated to their parent missions, the idea of a Union Mission Medical College. The obsession of training Indian women to take care of their sisters, drove Ida from the time she trained Salomi to be her first clinical assistant in 1900. It progressed to the start of the compounders training in 1903 and later to find helpers for Mrs. Gnanambal., It led to the informal training of local girls as nurses to look after the patients in the Mary Taber Schell Hospital The Nursing School with Delia Houghton in 1909 took birth until its culmination in the first class of the Union Mission Medical School for Women, Vellore in 1918.

The magnetism to this drive to educate Indian women to help their sisters was the personality of Ida. She was able to inspire all who came in contact with her,to share her dream and work with her. Salomi, an unschooled household helper who was trained by her became one of the loyal matrons of the Hospital on the Town Campus at Thottapalayam. Gertrud Dodd who gave up her life of comfort and luxury in New York to share Ida's life at Vellore and use her wealth for crucial development at Vellore.Mrs. Henry W. (Lucy) Peabody who caught Ida's vision for the medical college and worked for the rest of her life to raise funds from American women to support the health of Indian women,.All of them were wholly inspired by Ida and committed themselves to her vision wholeheartedly The role of her mother Mrs. Sophia Scudder, who while mourning the death of her beloved husband, gently supported and guided her daughter in all that she did for more than a quarter of a century.This is seldom recollected. A key person in the whole story is Colonel Bryson, the Surgeon General in Madras, who gave permission,knowing that on the ground at Vellore there was virtually nothing, but trusting that God would provide to His handmaiden. Yes, indeed, God had shown training as the right priority in India to Ida Sophia Scudder.She followed the light and inspired others to join her in the task to build a part of the Kingdom of God on land.

Chapter 4

Union Missionary Medical School for Women, Vellore 1918 – 1942

Dr. Ida Sophia Scudder, Dr. Jessie Findlay,
Ms. Gertrude Dodd

The Students 1918 to 1937

On Friday, 24th March 1922, was the graduation of the students, selected by Aunt Ida in July 1918, the Class of 1918, which was held at Vellore. Fourteen graduates were already selected to work in different places who gathered for this memorable event. The four years in Vellore with their Aunt Ida and other teachers had formed them into professionals who could work independently and serve their fellow men. These four years are best described in the words of Miss Lizzie Borges, who was to work at the American Evangelical Lutheran Mission Hospital in Guntur, now in Andhra Pradesh.

"We are glad to welcome you to our final class day exercises and it is my privilege to give you something of the History of our Class.

Looking back over the past four years, we realise the honour which is ours, as the first students of Vellore Medical School, an honour which none can ever share with us. Twenty–five years hence, when we come back to class day and closing exercises, we will say to the students 'We were present when this College was opened'.

August 12th 1918 – a day of great vision and inspiration. The ceremony was conducted by His Excellency Lord Pentland and it took place at the bungalow on Officer's Lines, which we are still using as a hostel and which bears his name.

In his opening speech, he said that he admires the courage and enthusiasm with which the Medical School Committee had approached the problems of establishing a Christian Medical College for Women of South India. He spoke of the great need for such a school and said that the Madras Government welcomed the proposal of the Committee to establish this School in Vellore and was glad to extend to it financial assistance.

We also had with us on that occasion Col. Bryson, whom we are glad to see with us here today again. He spoke of the urgency of the need for medical aid through the thousands of Indian villages and read an extract from a letter from one of his former students showing the pioneering work he was doing. He spoke of the honour which is ours as the first students of this School and also of the responsibility of setting the standard by which the Vellore Medical School will be judged in the future – that in our hands rests the reputation of our alma mater – these truths we are beginning to realise.

The college was opened with a class of eighteen students, and these were accommodated in the two bungalows that we still hold on Officers' Line. As our numbers increased, a third bungalow across the road was added the following year. This year, we have been happy with this, the first of new college buildings – the Fille Brown Hostel – although twenty of the new students are still living in the Pentland bungalow.

With the growth and development,college sports and activities have been hard to keep up with. Next year, the student body are looking forward to all being together in this compound.

The lectures were held in classrooms at the Voorhees College in the mornings and in the various bungalows' verandahs in the afternoon. We remember well our first lecture in Anatomy, with its long, jaw–breaking words. But our kind and painstaking Dr. Scudder soon simplified it and reminded us that we had only to learn one thing at a time, which led us to believe that the course was an easy one. But lo and behold! This idea was changed a few days later when we were marched to the dissection room. We were indeed frightened and horrified and, for many days and nights, were pursued by delusions of persecution.

During the first year, four of our classmates left us, one giving up the study for matrimony. Another dropped out the second year, but the remaining thirteen have moved on bravely with the addition of one this year. We hope we are now at last on the verge of full–fledged Medical Practitioners.

Our staff of professors have been steadily growing. There have been numerous changes during the four years. Dr. Scudder, our beloved Principal has been with us and our best friend all the way through. In our first year, we had Dr. Kinnaman, Miss Samuel and Mr. Harris of Voorhees College. The following year, Dr. Macphail was added to our number. This lasted for a year, when both she and Dr. Kinnaman left us and their places were taken by Dr. Findlay. During our third year too, Dr. Warnshuis, Dr. Scott and Miss Petrie were added to the list of staff members.

In the last year, Dr.J. Findlay had to leave us to fulfil an agreement made before coming to us to return to the Canadian Baptist Mission for one year. Dr. Griscom generously gave us her services and the benefit of her wide experience and knowledge. She has now left for her home in America. Miss Mitcheson was our house–mother during the first year. The following year, her place was taken by Miss Mann who has, we feel, always done her best to make our college life homely and to encourage and comfort us when we are tired. Although few in number, in our first year, our activities were many.

The Student Association began with Miss Joshua as the first President. During the second year, when 28 new students were added to our ranks, the Association took on new duties and committees were organised for sports, entertainment and self–government. These have added much to the school spirit. We have had basketball, volleyball, badminton tournaments, picnics and moonlight dinners. The hard grind was sometimes lightened by mock trials to impress upon our minds the court proceedings in Medical Jurisprudence; weekly visits to village dispensaries were done, where the hygiene and sanitation of the village were looked into – if having a picnic the Filter Reservoir Beds was an ideal one We can assure you that the sham caesarean section, where you become your own patient, and this enactment, was not only a good sport but profitable. Our Saturday afternoons will always remain in our memories – they are our free hours – a fact well known to certain of our visitors. Punctually at the stroke of 12 noon, our first visitor makes his appearance with a basket of tempting fruits. Next, comes the hawker with an array of colours in attires and a continual haggling of prices goes on. The cobbler and the tailor walk in with his bundle of valuables. Then comes the stately dhoby with his long train of loaded donkeys, and at times, a juggler drowns us with shrieking music. Saturday afternoon – mark you – is our free time. On Saturday nights, too, latecomers have been known to find their beds missing or occupied by a dummy.

The YWCA Student Secretary, Miss Wilson, visited us in our second year and organised a student branch of the YWCA, which has done much to stimulate our religious life during our College days. We have visits from many YWCA leaders and the yearly conferences where students from many colleges meet together for a common purpose, face the same problems, and enjoy the same recreational activities, which affords us an opportunity for rare Christian fellowships that will never be forgotten. It has been a privilege to meet, as a body of students, many distinguished visitors who have come to Vellore to see our College (A long list of visitors follow); the Acting Surgeon General Lieut. Col. Symmonds was here this year and presented the Gold Medal for highest proficiency in Anatomy in the Madras Presidency to Miss Kamala Israel (Class of 1919).

And now, as we leave this Institution and take up our work in the various parts of this great land, we will always strive to remember as we go in and out among our patients that our success or failure will be shared by our College though many a time we are tempted to be slack. We will remember that the people watching us will say, "She was trained at Vellore,' We will do our best to make that name the very highest in unselfish service to the needy women of India."

The list of the 14 graduates of 1922 (the Class of 1918) and the hospitals they were to work in shows their diversity and the spread of their services all over southern India and abroad:

Miss Krupa Abraham, Buscah, Arabia

Miss Jessilet Asirvatham, ABM Hospital, Pithapuram Miss Lizzie Borges, AELM Hospital Guntur

Miss Navamani David, AMM Hospital, Wadi, Southern Maharashtra.

Miss Lucy Devavaram, Schell Hospital, Vellore.

Miss Ebenezer Gnanamuthu, Rainy Hospital, Madras. Miss Dhanam Joshua, AELM Hospital, Guntur.

Miss Elizabeth Julian, Schell Hospital, Vellore

Miss Cecilia Lawrence, CEZM Hospital, Bangalore.

Miss Sophie Muthalamuthu, AM Hospital, Madurai.

Miss Thai Samuel, Government Hospital, Quilon, Travancore

Miss Kanagam Stevens, Lyles Hospital, Madanapalle.

Mrs. A. Thomas, Alwaye, Travancore

Over 400 young girls, who had completed high school, were admitted in the twenty classes from 1918 to 1937. Not all of them graduated and dropouts were regrettably 10 to 15% each year. The reasons for such discontinuation from medical studies were usually the decision by a student that she did not want or could not continue to study, chronic illnesses (e.g. tuberculosis) or a decision by the faculty that the student could not cope with the required academic rigour. The annual reports of the principal were available. It recorded the number and reasons why students dropped out of the course each year. Unfortunately, they are not available for several of the years making it difficult to analyse the cause for the high dropout rates, a phenomenon not seen nowadays. It was not an easy decision to let a student go and Aunt Ida and her faculty agonised over each drop out, knowing that strict academic accountability was essential to maintain high standards.

The limited faculty and clinical material at Schell Hospital (women and children only) forced Aunt Ida to recruit a variety of helpers to supplement the teaching. The clinical staff of the Government Pentland Hospital at Vellore, who had co-operated with her in providing anaesthesia to patients operated at the Schell Hospital, willingly helped in clinical teaching and provided access to male patients and their problems. The students spent two weeks each year with Dr. Frimodt Mueller at the Arogyavaram Tuberculosis Sanatorium at Madanapalle about a hundred kilometres away, for special training in tuberculosis and chest diseases. They also were taught by Dr. Cochrane at the Leprosy Hospital at Chingelpet. Most importantly, additional training in Obstetrics was provided at several mission hospitals in southern India where ultimately many of these graduates would work. Of course, the faculty of the Voorhees College who taught Physics and Chemistry were considered an integral part of the Medical School.

From rented bungalows on Officers' Line to the Rachel Fillebrown Hostel built for the Nurses on the Town Campus at Thottapalayam and finally to the beautiful, purpose–built college buildings at the Hill Campus at Bagayam in 1932, the students resided in a variety of progressively improving accommodation. The presence of dedicated house–mothers and the keen involvement of all faculty in their development were key factors in the transformation of the students. To these early students, Ida was truly an Aunt with special Tuesday evening Bible classes, involvement in all non–curricular activities and constant exhortations for academic excellence. The girls on arrival at Vellore were young, around eighteen years, Sixth Form (School Final) completed or graduated, shy and from protected backgrounds, timidly venturing on a career about which they knew little. The time with Aunt Ida and her colleagues in the Christian residential atmosphere of the School transformed them to confident doctors, who were prepared to face the challenge of helping their fellow women. This process of transformation of young boys and girls to confident health professionals is still the hallmark of Vellore. This tradition established by Aunt Ida and her early colleagues is continued by their students and successors.

The Faculty

The closing exercise report of 1922 also lists the then available faculty.

Miss Ida S Scudder, MD, Principal & Lecturer in Surgery and Gynaecology

Mrs. LC Warnshuis, MBChB, Lecturer in Medicine and Hygiene Miss MW Griscom, MD, Lecturer in Obstetrics

Miss E Findlay MD, Lecturer in Physiology

Miss KB Scott, MD, Lecturer in Anatomy and Physiology Miss JJ Petrie, MPS, Lecturer in Chemistry and Materia Medica

Miss MJ Samuel, LMP, Lecturer in Osteology and Dissecting Demonstrator

Miss G Dodd, Bursar

Mrs. JD Mann, Housemother

All the faculty were members of the Senatus, a committee, which helped the Principal run the School and the Mary Taber Schell Hospital, after it was handed over by the American Arcot Mission in 1923. The first Senatus in 1918 was Aunt Ida, Miss Dodd and Dr. MJ Samuel, the first Indian doctor to join the faculty, a Diplomate from Ludhiana. Every newcomer to the faculty, most of whom were missionary lady doctors, immediately became members of the Senatus. They would discuss all matters that affected the life and academics in the School and their recommendations, where policy was involved, would be presented to the Council by the Principal.

The 20th anniversary of the School was celebrated in February 1938, shortly after admissions to the LMP course were cancelled by the government. During the twenty years, in addition to several short term missionaries, Dr. Jessie Findlay (1920), Dr. Carol E Jameson (1923) Miss Treva Marshall (1925), Dr. HM Smith (1925), Dr. A Degenring (1925), Dr. Epps (1925), Dr. Pauline Jeffrey (1927), Dr. MD Graham (1929), Dr. Ida B Scudder (1931), Dr. Dorothy Jefferson (1935) and Dr. Bernadine Siebers (De Valois) served the School for five years or more. All of them had the basic equivalent of the MBBS degree and none had any postgraduate qualification. In 1938, when the School had to transform to the MBBS granting College, several faculty (Drs. Jameson, Graham, Ida B, Jefferson and newly joined Bernadine Siebers) were given study leave to obtain postgraduate degrees or diplomas that would qualify them to be on the University recognised faculty of the College.

Indian doctors also served the School from the beginning. Dr. (Miss) MJ Samuel, LMP from Ludhiana, was the first colleague of Aunt Ida, helping her teach Anatomy for over five years from 1918. From most graduating classes, at least two stayed on for a year as interns to refine their clinical skills and help carry the work load of the Hospital. Three of the LMP graduates, Ebenezer Gnanamuthu (Class of 1918, Dr. (Mrs.) Thomas), Kamala Israel (Class of 1919, Dr. (Mrs.) KI Vythilingam) and Miriam Manuel (1927), worked in mission hospitals for a short while and returned to work in the School. After a period, they were given study leave to do the short MBBS course in Madras. They were supported for postgraduate training when University affiliation became mandatory and joined the faculty. There were at least ten other Indian doctors who worked at the School during this time for short periods in Anatomy, Bacteriology and Pathology. The accepted faculty tradition was that in addition to your primary teaching responsibility, clinical work at the Hospital was a requisite, including regular participation in the outreach clinics – the roadside.

Dr. Jessie Findlay joined Aunt Ida at Vellore in 1920 and worked in the School till 1942. She was totally committed to Aunt Ida's vision of education for Indian women, and was her trusted colleague. Her name is missing in the list of faculty at the graduation of the Class of 1918 as she had taken a year off to fulfil an earlier commitment to serve the Canadian Baptist Hospital run by her supporting Mission. She was appointed as Vice-principal in 1924 and was also the Head of the Surgical Department of the School and Hospital. During all occasions, Aunt Ida was on furlough, she was the acting Principal (for a total of over 5 years). She was fully involved with the students and actually was the author(composer) of the College Song and the *Alma Mater*,which is still cherished by the College nearly a hundred years later. At the time of transition to the MBBS College, Dr. Findlay was the acting Principal as Aunt Ida was on furlough in the USA to raise funds. While several of her colleagues went abroad to obtain higher qualifications, Dr. Findlay felt that she was too old for that and when Dr. Cochrane joined the College, she quietly handed over her administrative responsibilities to him and served in her Mission's Hospital in India, for another five years. Truly, a person committed to women's health in India and totally inspired by Aunt Ida's vision of educating young Indian women to help their sisters, she was a dedicated Christian, a skillful surgeon and an astute administrator. The story of the Missionary Medical School for Women would have been different if she had not stood shoulder to shoulder with Aunt Ida in those early, difficult, formative years. CMCV recognises her by naming one of the four houses the students are divided into as Findlay House. I truly wonder if this was a sufficient commemoration?

Dr. Carol E Jameson was working at the Mayo Clinic when she came in contact with Aunt Ida on her promotional furlough 1922 to 1923. She was a young doctor with a brilliant career ahead of her and the Mayo brothers had already in their mind selected her to be on their faculty. Inspired by Aunt Ida, she decided to come to teach and work in Vellore. The Mayo Clinic offered her a faculty position but she did not waver in her decision. Her introduction to India was on her first roadside clinic within 24 hours of her arrival. Thrown into the swimming pool to learn swimming!

Her inspiring autobiography *"Be Thou My Vision"* published by CMCV is a tribute to her and a must read. Whenever Dr. Jessie was the Acting Principal, Dr. Carol was acting Vice-Principal. She served as acting Principal and later as acting Director. In addition to being elected FACS, she passed the FRCS in Canada to be eligible to teach MBBS students. Despite the examination being on General Surgery and all her experience at Vellore in Gynaecology, she passed at the first attempt and promptly returned to Vellore. Her journey from America to India during the Second World War was an adventure where she was stuck in Africa and ultimately hitched a ride with the Air Force to Delhi and took a train to Vellore arriving back on the day the College started in July 1942.

Treva Marshall was a student of dietetics in 1922, when she heard Aunt Ida speak about the needs for the women in India and the College. She tried to meet Ida repeatedly, but failed. Later, she got a message from Aunt Ida that Vellore needed a dietician and happily decided to complete her training before going there. Six months later, she got another message that the need for an X-ray technician was greater. Responding to this call, she took a further year of training and reached Vellore in 1925. Her services were used both to teach dietetics to the students and for diagnostic X-ray work, once the first major equipment was established, But she found her real role asa house- mother for the medical students of the School and later the College. In between, she also served for many years as the Deputy Council

Secretary for the Association and Council. Miss Marshall was the live wire that energised campus life at Bagayam and made the Women Students Hostel a home away from home. During her nearly four decades of service at Vellore, she was the prime force that welcomed new students, women initially and then the men when they were admitted and ensured that student traditions established over the years continued and were built upon.

Dr. Ida Belle Sophia Scudder (known to all who loved her as Ida B) was the daughter of Aunt Ida's brother Lewis Weld Scudder, a Pastor. Ida B grew up adoring her aunt whom she met on occasional furloughs to the US.She followed her footsteps at the Mount Holyoake Academy, went through four years of college and joined the Women's Medical College in Philadelphia, graduating in June, 1929. She spent a year as an Intern at the Albany Medical College and worked as a Resident in several hospitals and decided to go as a missionary to work with her aunt at Vellore. She arrived in India in April 1931 and was doing language school at Kodaikanal. She was called to Vellore and was put in charge of the Eye and ENT Department as Dr. Pauline Jeffrey who looked after it had to leave due to ill health. After a year, she had to take over the Medical Department as the doctor in charge was going on furlough! Ida B felt unqualified for both these responsibilities but tried to do her best. She was then asked to work with Carol Jameson in the Obstetric Department.

The tribute Aunt Ida paid to her staff in her Principal's report of 1938:

"I want to pay a loving tribute to our present splendid staff. Everymember has carried on their work in the most praise worthy way– forgetful of self and of fatigue– putting everything personal aside and giving themselves wholeheartedly and lovingly to the work in hand. All have carried far too heavy burdens – without a murmur. There has been love, loyalty, unity, and co-operation in the staff, making hard things easy. The Spirit of Christ has been in our midst and we thank Him for His continued blessing."

The continuation of this spirit by the staff of succeeding generations defines CMCV.

The Infrastructure

Along with increasing numbers of students and graduates, the clinical work load also increased. It became clear that the Mary Taber Schell Hospital originally planned for 50 patients was inadequate to meet the requirements of the growing Medical School. The Board in New York had agreed even before the Medical School started and realised that more facilities were needed for clinical work. One acre in the centre of the town, next to the Jutka Stand formed the nucleus of the Town Campus, which over the next 20 years became the centre of clinical activity. The building projects started in 1918, as money was being collected for the School. The government gave a matching grant of five lakhs of rupees over a five–year period for construction and purchase of land. The School at this time had three properties, the original Mary Taber Schell Campus, across the road from the Arcot Mission's Voorhees College Campus, the Town Campus on Arcot road, renamed Ida S Scudder road many years later, next to the Jutka Stand in the Thottapalayam area of town and the Hill Campus of about 200 acres, south of the Hill demarcating the southern extent of the town on the Arni road about six kilometres from the other two campuses. Aunt

Ida's original idea was that the Town Campus would primarily be an out-patient clinic and that the main Hospital and Medical College would be at the large Hill Campus.

Construction progressed on the Town Campus with the Cole dispensary, the Chapel which would be a focal point of all the buildings and a big bungalow where Aunt Ida and her family as well as other doctors would stay. Money was initally collected from America.

By the tireless efforts of Mrs. Peabody, work began on the Rachel Fillebrown hostel for nurses. As the increase of in-patients overwhelmed the limited accommodation at Schell, the decision to build additional wards and an out-patient facility on this campus was inevitable. Rev. Rottschaefer, the American Arcot Missionary in charge of the Katpady Industrial Institute, was an amateur architect and a skilled civil engineer. From the beginning, the Council agreed that he would plan and build all that was needed for the School. Their arrangement was unusual but practical. Aunt Ida and the other faculty would define their requirements for construction and work with Rev. Rottschaefer to develop plans for the buildings. These plans would be presented to the Council and after the plans and estimates were approved, the Treasurer, who held all the money sent from the New York Office for capital expenditure, would advance necessary amounts to him. Once the construction was completed, the quantity of work would be measured and the cost would be decided as per Government Public Works Department (PWD) rates, 5% would be added to defray Rev. Rottschaefer's costs and the account would be settled. This rather unusual arrangement was approved by the Council. They found that consistently the work was completed under the estimated amount and that the quality of the work was excellent. As time went on, they found that additional floors could safely be built on the foundations originally laid for one or two floors. Almost 80 years later, knocking down the Nurses Hostel built by Rev. Rottschaefer to build the Centenary block took almost three times more than the estimated time as it was built for the ages!

The Board in New York, several of the faculty at Vellore, and members of the Council pointed out the logistic difficulties and increased costs of having several campuses relatively far apart and suggested that the Institution should be built only on the Town Campus. It was also pointed out that a hospital far outside the town would present difficulties for the patient to access. In fact,during Aunt Ida's furlough in 1922–23, the Council passed a resolution that the entire Institution should be built on the Town Campus, but decided to keep the resolution on hold till she returned and could present her arguments to the Council in person. After detailed discussions, it was finally decided that all clinical facilities, out –patients, wards and nurses accommodation would be built on the Town Campus, but the Medical School and faculty accommodation would be built at the Hill Campus. The vote in favour of clinical facilities in town was seventeen to one, while vote for building the School at the Hill Campus was eleven to seven. The feelings for and against were strong and this is the only resolution where the actual names of those who voted for and against is recorded in the Minutes. It was also decided that the work at the Town Campus should be completed before any work started at the Hill Campus. In spite of this resolution, the discussion continued till construction at the Hill Campus started in 1928, after the facilities in town were formally inaugurated by the Governor in

Madras. If they had stalled till all construction activity on the Town Campus were done they would still be waiting today!

Life in the Missionary Medical School for Women, Vellore

The students of the First Batch of 1918, were specially privileged. Aunt Ida was their teacher for all the first –year subjects except Chemistry taught by the Voorhees College next door. In addition to Physiology, Anatomy and Chemistry, they worked from the beginning in the Mary Taber Schell Hospital, beside her imbibing her special empathy for patients. Her constant admonitions to strive for excellence ensured that all of them passed the first–year examination held in Madras and the School topped the State in the results, a position they held for most years of the LMP programme. Every week, two intern students would go for the outreach clinics with Aunt Ida, a valuable training opportunity with real life situations and learn the existing realities of life in Indian villages. With an elected student President and other responsible office bearers, students also learnt about self–governance and responsibility with their committees. They were encouraged to take part in games and extracurricular activities. The Young Women's Christian Association and the Student Christian Movement supplemented the spiritual nourishment provided by Aunt Ida and the faculty. Aunt Ida was very much their guide, philosopher and friend during their four years to graduation. The fact that all fourteen of them passed the final examination, whereas the pass percentage in other Schools in the Presidency was around 25%. This was solely due to the dynamic and inspiring leadership and the commitment and hard work of the girls and faculty.

Aunt Ida was clear that caring for the patients should not be confined just to the Hospital. She started her day, in the early years, by house visits to the homes of patients of whom, she knew would not come to the Hospital. The caste system and social norms precluded many of the well–to–do families sending their women to the Hospital. She had realised early that she also was called to take medical care to the villages surrounding Vellore and started a clinic at Gudiyattam about 30 km to the west of Vellore. With the increase of personnel in the School and addition of cars and ambulances to the original Peugeot and Model–T Ford, the outreach programme increased and at its height there were five roadside clinics, one on each day of the week. This was an important activity of the Institution and provided an excellent learning opportunity for students. Community based work was a priority at Vellore from its inception and this commitment grew with the years.

The increase in the amount and complexity of the clinical work at the Hospital was steady. All medically qualified faculty despite their title as Lecturer in whatever nonclinical subject, were also involved in–patient care. All were residents on the campus and were always at all times available.

They worked twenty four hours if work demanded. Their students were also involved in this work. Aunt Ida delighted in demonstrating surgery to the students and each case was seen as an opportunity for training. A clinical laboratory started by Dr. Petrie with manual techniques enhanced the diagnostic skills of the clinicians. A simple X–ray machine, installed by the mid–twenties under the supervision of Miss Marshall was upgraded in the mid–thirties and Ida B was requested to have special training in both diagnostic radiology and in radiation therapy.

The first cobalt tele–radiotherapy machine was installed by the time she returned after training and its services were in great demand. All faculty accepted excellence, in–patient care and empathy with them which was the best way to witness their faith.

The increasing number of patients, the roadside outreach programme –expanding to five days a week, a breakthrough in leprosy therapy with Chaulmoogra oil injections and Aunt Ida's innovation for the repair of vesico–vaginal fistulas making many women regain normal lives were some of the highlights of the clinical work during this period. It was not all work but plenty of joy at the school. Evenings, picnics and moonlight dinners with the students, detailed reports from graduates from mission hospitals all over the country and the companionship of the faculty and encouragement and support of the Council and the Governing Boards were just rewards for all at Vellore. All this and more, in the presence of a constant stream of visitors, each treated as a VIP by Aunt Ida to see the pioneering work at Vellore.

Life was not easy at the School. Electricity was connected at Schell and the Town Campus only by 1927. Air conditioning was unknown on the campus and the staff, especially the expatriates who had to adapt to working in temperatures unknown to them before they arrived in Vellore. All the expatriates staff looked forward to a break at a hill station usually in summer. If they went for the break to Kodaikanal, the hospitality of Aunt Ida's hilltop house was available to them. All expatriate staff had to have lessons in Tamil and while it was enough to communicate with patients, none of them became Tamil scholars! Staff service rules were put in place and salary scales were established for Indian staff. The missionary staff including Aunt Ida, were paid Rs. 200/– per month and it did not change during the first 20 years of the School. A contributory provident fund was set up initially for the faculty and later extended to cover all the confirmed staff. This fund was approved by the Income Tax Department.

Aunt Ida and especially her friend, Annie Hancock, working as an evangelist with women in Vellore, were particularly interested in improving the societal status of women. Their ideas fitted in with the social changes sweeping over India with the call for independence under the leadership of Mahatma Gandhi. In fact, he visited Vellore in 1926 and came to the Hospital to address the staff and students, even though they did not accept his call to change the uniform to Khadi cloth! The School worked very closely with the British Government of the then Madras Presidency. Visits from the Governors of Madras, invitation to Aunt Ida and others for official functions in Madras, grants for the support of students and for buildings in the Town Campus showed this close relationship. While winds of political turmoil were sweeping through the country, the School was a place of tranquillity where Indians and people from overseas worked together in the Spirit of Christ for a common goal, the health of women and children of India.

Tragedies personally affecting Aunt Ida, also occurred during this period. Annie Hancock, devoted worker for women's empowerment and ardent preacher of the Gospel to the women of Vellore, contracted Cholera and died in Vellore in 1924, a month before she was due to leave on furlough. She became a close companion and friend of Aunt Ida at Mount Holyoke and was determined to accompany her to Vellore years later when she was preparing to be a missionary doctor.

The board was reluctant to support her but Miss Dodd sponsored her to accompany Aunt Ida at the Arcot Mission in Vellore as an evangelist for women. Her quiet advocacy resulted in the Women's Club at Vellore,. It played a socially transforming role as a centre where women could gather and play games like tennis together and also discuss issues of mutual interest. She was a constant support to Ida in her quiet way and had much influenced the emancipation of women in Vellore.

An equally great loss was that of Mrs. Sophia Scudder, Aunt Ida's mother. In 1925 at the age of 84, her health started to fail. She had come to India as a young bride in 1860 and went back for the first time 17 years later with her five children. The call of the mission work brought Dr. John Scudder back to India, three years later,when his health had improved but she stayed back for another two years with the children and then joined her husband. Soon after Aunt Ida came back to work with her father, he died. Mrs. John Scudder was the chief guide, philosopher and strength to Aunt Ida as she struggled to gain acceptance as a woman doctor, build up the Schell Hospital and dreamt of starting the Medical College for women. There are anecdotes that in the early years, the women who came for treatment insisted that she look after them rather than the young girl! As news of Mrs. John Scudder's ill health spread through the town, crowds thronged to see her. She died on 30 August 1925, after 64 years of service in India. Her death was a great loss to the people.

Conclusion

Ida Sophia Scudder was born in India in December 1870, and on her first trip back to America, she declared that she would never be 'another Scudder Missionary' committed to work in India. God confronted her with the challenge of women's health in India, and she agonised and accepted the challenge. At the age of 30, she came back to India as a qualified doctor looking forward to working with her father and learning the ropes of working in India. The tragic loss of her father to cancer did not prevent her from starting her work and realising that training Indian girls to work as health professionals would maximise her impact on women's health. Beginning with the training of compounders and nurses she was able to establish the Union Missionary Medical School for Women, awarding the licentiate diploma and train almost 300 young women of India to be skilled and dedicated doctors as well as many nurses. Her unique ability was to transmit the vision that motivated her to many who came in contact with her, Jessie Findlay, Ida B Scudder, Treva Marshall, MD Graham, Dorothy Jefferson, Carole Jameson and many other missionary women doctors received the call and played key roles in the development of women's medical education. Mrs. Henry Peabody and many others with the Board in New York, played a key supporting role. Above all others, Miss Margaret Dodd, a wealthy New York socialite used her wealth and position to make Ida's dreams a reality. Aunt Ida was clear she was

The traditions that uphold CMCV today were established during the 20 years of the Union Missionary Medical School for Women. When the Licentiate programme was abolished by the State government, Vellore was offered the chance to upgrade to the full MBBS degree–granting status. This was a huge challenge to Aunt Ida and her team and the Council and Board that administered the Institution. How they faced and resolved this major challenge is the story of the next chapter.

Chapter 5

The Council, The Board and the Road to MBBS

Dr. Ida S Scudder, Dr. Jessie Findlay, and Dr. Chone Oliver

The mission of an inspired and charismatic visionary can be accomplished only if she is able to enthuse a group of fellow workers to share the vision, money is available to support the work and a responsive governance and administrative machinery guides it forward. Aunt Ida was fortunate that all three requisites for her vision to be realised were available. Starting with two colleagues in 1918, she was able to draw an able and committed team to work with her to nurture the students. All the missions working in southern India were her enthusiastic supporters prepared to share medical missionaries to work with her. The missions also registered a society in India, and their parent bodies in the USA and UK formed boards to support Ida's work. The strategies and practices established by this early and inspired governance are a lasting legacy for CMCV.

Governance and Administration

Ida Scudder was a missionary of the American Arcot Mission of the Reformed Church in America, started by the Scudder brothers in 1855, with headquarters in Vellore and a Mission Board in New York. Heavily involved in education, industrial training and a hospital in Ranipet, the Mission was farsighted and realised that the venture in medical education that Ida started went much beyond the confines of the American Arcot Mission. It was an ecumenical or as then called 'A Union' venture in which almost all the different missions at work in southern India were partners. It was essential that this was reflected in new systems of governance and administration for the school envisaged as an interdenominational institute.

Five American missions working in southern India registered an Association which was the legal owner of the school in India. They were the American Arcot Mission, the American Baptist Telugu Mission, the American Evangelical Lutheran Mission, the American Madura Mission and the Wesleyan Methodist Missionary Society. They were joined by the Danish Evangelical Lutheran Mission. The parent mission bodies formed a governing board for the school located in New York, under the leadership of the American Arcot Mission. A British Committee for the medical school in Vellore was established by 1922 with representation in the Association in India.

Two representatives from each of the missions in the Association formed a Council with powers to co-opt others. This Council was responsible for governance of the School subject to the final approval by the boards in New York and the UK. The boards were responsible to ensure necessary funds for the school. The Association in India and its Council had oversight of the way the school was run and for approving an annual budget, based on the working budget drafted by the Bursar and her faculty colleagues. The budget approved by the Council would be forwarded by the treasurer to the boards in the USA and the UK. The budget would have a list of expenditures and also show what the Medical School and the Hospital was expected to earn that year in India. In the early years, the income of the school was larger than that of the hospital. The vast majority of the patients were being treated free. An affordable tuition fee was charged to the students who also had to pay for their board. The Colonial Government provided a grant based on the number of students.

The President (Chair), Secretary and Treasurer of the Council were elected annually from the members of the Association. A Joint Secretary for the Council was selected from the faculty starting from 1926 to help the Council Secretary. There was faculty representation on the Council, the Principal, the Vice-principal, a Bursar appointed from the seventh generation faculty by the Council and a representative of the Senatus, serving as full voting members of the Council. All Council decisions and budgets approved by the Council were sent to the parent board for final approval so that necessary funds could be raised. An Executive Committee of the Chair, Secretary, Treasurer, Principal, Bursar, Joint Secretary and at least two other members of the Council was authorised to act on behalf of the Council in between meetings of the Council. The Council was only responsible for the governance of the school till 1922 when the Mary Taber Schell Hospital was transferred from the American Arcot Mission, the original mission through which A unt Ida came to India in 1900.

The earliest available printed Minutes of the Council is dated 4 and 5 August 1921, three years after the College was established. There are references to earlier Executive Committee and Council decisions, but these records are not available. It appears that August 1921 was the first printed Minutes as there is an item (Minute 11 of October 1922) authorising the payment of Rs. 32 and 10 Annas to the Secretary as cost of printing the Minutes of 1921 and 1922! The Council Minutes over the next 17 years record the growth and development of the School. It is a pity that these Minutes are incomplete and that in almost half the years the Principal's report is not available. The major concerns and challenges to the fledgling School are clear from the Council Minutes. Appointing suitable faculty, building essential infrastructure, economy in expenditure, student welfare, outreach programmes and the need to upgrade to a university–affiliated Medical College were the primary concerns of the Council. The Council shared Aunt Ida's vision to optimise the healthcare of Indian women and children as a means of preaching the Gospel.

The outstanding features of governance, which make CMCV an institution where faculty are proud and eager to serve, were all established by the Council of the Missionary Medical School for Women during these formative years. A key tradition established from the beginning was that the nitty–gritty of administration was the responsibility of the principal and faculty, the Council offering guidance and oversight from their collective wisdom. In addition to the two representatives from each of the Association members, the faculty were represented on the Council as full voting members participating in policy decisions. The majority of Council members were not faculty but almost all items that came up for decision and discussion were brought up through the Senatus by the Principal and the faculty. The Council would decide on policy but it was Aunt Ida and her colleagues who would actualise these decisions, a balance that is continued even now. Most key aspects of the life and functioning of CMCV today are the results of policies established in the 1920s by Aunt Ida and her Council. The Council Minutes referred below listing some of these key decisions are identified by the minute number, followed by a colon, the month of the meeting and the year of the meeting. The Council Minutes were initially numbered for each meeting, but from August 1927 they were sequentially numbered, the sequence continuing till now.

The appropriate faculty cadre for effective functioning of the Institution was determined by the Council based on requests developed and forwarded by the Senatus [Cl. 16(b):8– 1921]. The appointment, evaluation and disciplining of faculty [Cl. 16(c, d, e):8–1921], fixation of salary scales [16(l):8–1921] and appointment of Administrative Officers [Cl. 79:8–1928] were functions of the Council. Study leave for enhancing professional competence was initially encouraged during furlough of missionary staff, the Council paying the expenses. Study leave was granted in the interest of the Institution for obtaining academic degrees for missionary staff and later on for LMP graduates to upgrade to the MBBS degree and also for postgraduate qualification.

The Council passed a standing rule that all accounts must be professionally and externally audited before presentation to Council [Cl. 5:7–1922]. An equipment fund was created and Senatus was authorised to spend up to Rs. 5000/– from it without further reference to Council [Cl. 24:7–1922]. A very farsighted policy was the establishment of a Depreciation fund for replacement of equipment [Cl. 225:8–1933]. However, depreciation was not budgeted as an actual expenditure. Whenever money became available, for example the sale of an old vehicle, some amount would be put aside as depreciation to be used for replacement of equipment. Equally farsighted was the establishment of a contributory provident fund, initially only for the faculty but later extended to all confirmed staff. The contribution was one Anna in each Rupee of salary (6.25%) with an equal contribution from the Institution, managed by trustees appointed by the Council and recognised by the Income Tax Department (Cl. 39:2–1927). In addition to the Provident Fund, provision was also made for retirement benefits on a case by case basis for the faculty, co–operating with their supporting Missions. An example is Dr. Degenring, in charge of the Medical Department for over 15 years at the School was given a pension in association with her supporting mission.

All property was held in the name of the Association, and much of the land which was in Aunt Ida's name was transferred to the Association. The Council, which had a large number of co–opted members initially, ultimately decided that co–opted members should be limited in number to one–third of the number of Association members [Cl. 104:81929]. The Council–appointed a Building Committee [Cl. 26:8–1921], an external finance advisory committee [Cl. 31:8–1921], and Committees to review the Constitution and Staff service condition [Cl. 5:11–1923 and Cl. 8:11–1923]. It is remarkable that this structure of governance established in the early nineteen– twenties is virtually identical with the structure of the present Association and its Council. The critical difference is that only Indian Churches and Christian bodies are currently eligible for membership in the Association ensuring that CMCV is owned and administered as an Indian

Christian organisation. Representation of overseas mission bodies, especially the original founders of the School, continue as members of the Council.

Who were the visionaries setting this pattern? They were all missionaries working in missions in southern India who had been inspired by Aunt Ida's vision to train Indian women to treat their sisters and were keen to be her partners. Fourteen members were present at the meeting in August 1921 including four ordained pastors, six doctors and four others. Almost half of them were women. A significant co–opted member was Miss MacDougall, Principal of the Women's Christian College in Madras (now Chennai). This was one of the seven academic institutions in Asia, sponsored by the International Missionary Union for whom Mrs. Peabody initially raised three million dollars, a million of which was the share of CMCV. Rev. JS Chandler of the American Madura Mission was the President who chaired the Council in 1921 and Rev. LH Warnshuis of the American Arcot Mission was the Secretary. The Treasurer was Rev. FC Marquis and Miss Dodd was the Bursar selected from the faculty. The Council would meet at least twice a year,when the meeting usually lasted for a day at Vellore. The Executive Committee would meet at Chennai when necessary. The additional work of serving Vellore was happily borne by all as they were inspired by Aunt Ida's vision and it became part of their commitment to witnessing for Christ and building the Kingdom of God in India.

What was the role of the boards? The Board in New York had representatives from all the American Missions working in southern India. Many of the initial members of the Board actually had a personal commitment to Aunt Ida and were determined to do all that. Thereby making her vision a successful reality. An example was Mrs. Henry (Lucy) Peabody who had spent a day in 1913 at Vellore during which Aunt Ida shared her vision of training Indian women to care for the health of their sisters and their children. Inspired by this, she was primarily responsible for raising funds for the School through the Board. Aunt Ida and Miss Dodd worked with her on campaigns to raise funds during their furloughs in America. The boards also were on the lookout for lady doctors who would be challenged to go to Vellore and work shoulder to shoulder with Aunt Ida. Usually, the Board could count on the Mission Board of the Church to which the Doctor belonged to fund their travel and salaries. Much of the money was raised by $1 contributions by ordinary women who had heard Aunt Ida speaking in their churches. The UK Board functioned in much the same way although the finances raised by them were of a smaller order.

Finance

Money was essential to drive Aunt Ida's vision forward. Permission had been granted by the Mission Board to start the Medical School, expand the beds in the Mary Taber Schell Hospital to 100 by building four more wards and to purchase land in the middle of Vellore to put up a new dispensary in early 1914, but she was expected to raise the bulk of funds. During her furlough in the USA in 1914–15 she worked long and hard along with Mrs. Peabody to raise funds. She had the promise of a grant of up to 20,000 dollars from the Colonial Government in Madras if she could raise double that amount as matching funds. However, it was the height of the First World War and even though the USA was not at war then, the priorities were not for improving women's health in distant India. Mrs. Peabody and Aunt Ida with the Board managed to raise just enough to qualify for applying for the government grant.

Lucy Peabody and others on the Board in New York continued to try to raise funds for the Medical School, and they were promised from the Rockefeller Foundation a grant of a million dollars if they could raise two million for the several women's educational institutions in the Oriental East! The campaign started in real earnest, not only for the Medical School in Vellore but for six other educational institutions for women in south and east Asia, including the Women's Christian College in Madras. The deadline to raise the funds was 31 December 1922, and it was extended to 31 January 1923. Soon after the graduation of the first class of students in 1922, Aunt Ida and Miss Dodd left on furlough to join the campaign in the USA. Nine months of hard work by all still left them 50,000 short of two million as the deadline drew near. The Rockefeller offer was a million for raising two million and there was no fallback option if the amount raised was less than two million! On the last day, a lady that Mrs. Peabody had met a week earlier in California gave 50,000 dollars bringing the total collected to two million dollars, which the Rockefeller Foundation matched with another million. The share of Vellore was a million dollars. This was supplemented by a grant of five lakhs of rupees from the Colonial Government in Madras. Although this was a grant and not a loan, the School had to pledge all their property for 30 years with the Government, to guarantee that all that was promised would be fulfilled! The promises were more than fulfilled and the papers redeemed in due course.

The clinical work at Schell Hospital and academics in the School were in full flow. Salaries had to be paid, medicines purchased and vehicles fuelled! The Budget for the School for 1923–24 anticipated an income of Rs. 65620/– which included a Government grant of Rs. 16750/– at Rs. 250/– per year per student, tuition fees of Rs. 4080/– approximately Rs. 60/– per student and a Board contribution of Rs.44700/–. The actuals presented in the audited statement of accounts next year showed an income of Rs. 55001/– (Board Rs. 32830/–, Tuition fee Rs. 3894/–, and the government grant of Rs. 17500/–). The account was balanced by borrowing Rs. 11853/– from funds invested from savings in previous years. The Minutes recorded the necessity to pay this back in due course. The budgeted expenditure was Rs. 55052/– of which salaries was Rs. 43709/–. The actual expenditure for the School was 20% less at Rs. 44970/– of which Rs. 36139/– was for primarily faculty salaries. Nearly 12% of the expenditure (Rs.5527/–) was for conveyance, the roadside extension work and transport in different campuses.

The budgeted income of the Schell Hospital for Women for that year was Rs. 18800/– and expenditure was Rs. 23725/–. The actuals were close to the estimate, income Rs. 18272/– of which Rs. 8324/– was from patients and Rs. 8920/– was contributed by the Board and other donors. Staff salaries were Rs. 8698/– of the total expenditure of Rs. 24830/–. While Rs. 6122/– worth of drugs was used in the Hospital only Rs. 1622/– was collected from patients because most of the patients were treated free.

The total expenditure for the School and Hospital was Rs. 69800/–. Salaries were the major expenditure accounting for Rs. 44837/–. All salaries of mission personnel working in the School was shown in the budget accounting for the high proportion of salaries. The total earned from patients (Rs. 8324/–) and student fees was Rs. 12218/– clearly showing that the contribution by the boards (Rs. 41750/–) was the major income that sustained the work of Aunt Ida. A tariff for the beds and treatment was implemented only by the mid–thirties so that a larger income could be generated locally. However, the educational activities continued to be heavily subsidised as they are at present. The grant per student from the Colonial Government made a significant difference to the finances and made the whole enterprise viable. All capital expenses, especially for the buildings on the Town Campus were met by the Board in New York.

An average of 6500 to 7000 patients were seen each month, including those seen at the roadside extension work. About 190 patients were admitted each month as in–patients, many of them requiring surgery. While the patients seen as out–patients were expected to put something in the collection box, it was usually one paisa. The paisa was the smallest coin, with 192 making one rupee! The total collection from patients for the year was Rs. 8324/–. This included the voluntary contributions, charges for the few rooms they had for rich and upper caste patients and recoveries for medicines. The Rs. 1622/– received from patients for medicines contrasts with the expenditure for medicines of Rs. 6122/– for the year. Truly, the vast majority of the patients especially the ones seen on the outreach programmes, were seen free in the best tradition of Christian charity. The Missionary Medical School for Women was a very lean, but not a mean operation.

During this period, the funds received by the Treasurer for capital expenditure supported the purchase of additional land at the Town site, the heavy schedule of construction and scholarships disbursed to the students. The scholarships for the students supported their expenses other than tuition and played an important role in the viability of the School. Scholarship recipients were required to spend at least two years working in mission hospitals and signed a bond for that. Miss Dodd as Bursar, a responsibility she took on voluntarily, was responsible for the administration of the scholarships. She kept close contact with the students to ensure that they fulfilled their responsibility. The traditions of prudence, responsible spending and making every rupee count were established by Miss Gertrude Dodd, Aunt Ida and the faculty from the beginning of the Institution.

The Road to MBBS

The announcement by Aunt Ida inviting students to join the Missionary Medical School for Women in 1918 had made it clear that the intention was to start a Medical College leading to the MBBS degree from the Madras University, while initially students were to be admitted to the Diploma course. Aunt Ida was always keen to start the College, but none of the teachers including her had the minimum academic qualifications necessary to be considered as faculty by the University. Schell Hospital was primarily a women and children's hospital and male patients were seen mainly on the roadside outreach clinics. A full–fledged hospital catering to women, children and men, with appropriate infrastructure, laboratories and fully staffed and equipped departments was essential for recognition by the University. The infrastructure, faculty and finances for such a venture was beyond the means of the boards. The cost of transformation from the Diploma to MBBS was conservatively estimated to be of the order of US$ two million in 1928, about ten years after the Medical School was started. The service of the diploma graduates fulfilled the need of the missions for health personnel and they were valued wherever they served. The dream to start MBBS remained a dream for 20 years.

The first elected Indian Government in the Madras Presidency changed this situation at one stroke. On 17 October 1937, the Health Minister announced that students thereafter would only be admitted to the MBBS course and no further admissions for the Diploma would be permitted from the 1938–39 academic year. The two schools admitting students for the Diploma, a Government school in Madras and the Missionary Medical School for Women at Vellore, were offered the opportunity to upgrade to the MBBS programme. This opportunity for transition was welcomed by Aunt Ida and the Council in India, but for four long years no more new students could be admitted while Vellore and the boards struggled to find the human resources and finance to satisfy the minimum requirements for university recognition.

Another major change had been proposed to the Council in 1936. Dr. Chone Oliver, the then Secretary of the Christian Medical Association of India (CMAI) acting on a suggestion from the National Christian Council of India (NCCI) that it was essential to have an Indian Christian Medical College training both women and men for the MBBS degree, initiated a discussion, requesting Aunt Ida and the Council to take up this challenge. The NCCI had explored the possibility of starting such a college in Allahabad, possibly in association with the Agricultural Institute and had found that financially and in terms of the required human resources, it was not feasible. Among the three Christian medical schools in India at that time, their first choice was to request Vellore to start such a programme. The Council reportedly discussed this proposition in August 1936 (the minutes of this meeting are not available) and in Cl 316:8–1936 appointed a Committee to consider the options further (CL 316: 8–1936). Since that Committee did not meet due to a variety of issues, the Council in February 1937 (CL 335: 2–1938) expanded the Committee with a mandate to report back at the next meeting. Cl 357(b):8–1938 reads as follows:

"357 (b) "Minute "335 (b) "Report "of "Committee "on "Amalgamation."

The Secretary read the report of the Committee after which the Chairman of the Committee made a statement outlining most recent developments, both with respect to amalgamation with the proposed Union Christian Medical College, and the desirability to raise our school to the M.B.B.S. College grade. After long consideration it was:

Resolved to put on Record :

1. We believe that the Christian Church has a contribution to make to the Medical Training of Women in India which no other agency can make.

2. It was with a view to making this contribution effectively that Vellore College was founded.

3. It is now clear that the present grade of education does not satisfy those who receive it. It is clear also that we may at any time be faced with the abolition of the L.M.P. Course. (The LMP had already been abolished by the Government by the time this resolution was passed, and no student had been admitted at Vellore for the academic year 1938–39).

4. We believe that it must be the will of God that the specific Christian contribution to medical education shall continue to be made.

5. Although therefore we fully realise the difficulties in the way we feel compelled at once to prepare the way for raising the College to the M.B. Standard (a) by examining carefully the financial implications of this step, (b) by studying the immediate actions to be taken to raise the existing staff and equipment to the requirements of the higher standard."

Although the Committee was to consider amalgamation with the NCCI–CMAI proposed Union Christian Medical College, the resolutions refer only to upgrading the diploma course to MBBS and reiterates their commitment to medical training for women. There were sharp differences of opinion even in the Council about considering admitting men to the School. Aunt Ida saw the wisdom and necessity of a coeducational MBBS course, which would have the support of the NCCI and the entire medical missionary community in India, but also appreciated the validity of the opinion of those who felt that they were primarily called to help the women of India. Mrs. Peabody and others on the Board in New York, responsible for raising much of the money for the School went so far as to say that if men were to be admitted, all the money collected would have to be refunded as otherwise it would have been collected under false pretences! Aunt Ida's quarter century of friendship with Mrs. Peabody was under threat. Mrs. Peabody considered even the thought that the College may admit men a complete betrayal of all she and Ida had worked for nearly three decades. Aunt Ida's dilemma was to discern whether God was calling her to a wider new vision or she should have no vision other than the original.

Avoiding a direct commitment to admitting men, the Council went ahead with preparation for applying to the University for affiliation for the MBBS course. In January 1939, study leave was granted to eight faculty so that they could obtain British or Canadian postgraduate degrees that would be recognised by the University (CL412: 1–1939). The Council also requested the boards for permission to apply to the University for affiliation for the MBBS course (CL 413: 1–1939). That August, Council decided that all undesignated funds received for the School should be kept for new buildings and staff training for the University recognition, even if it was designated for the endowment for supporting the Institution (CL 435: 8–1939). Council also resolved to recommend to the boards that Aunt Ida and Miss Dodd, who were to go on furlough, should return to the School as Principal and Registrar on completion of the furlough, in spite of the fact that they would both be over 70 years of age (Cl 431: 8–1939). Aunt Ida and Miss Dodd were scheduled to go on furlough to the UK and USA primarily to raise funds for the changeover to MBBS in 1939, but on the eve of their departure the Second World War broke out and their plans had to be cancelled.

The Council in March 1940 (Cl 444:2–1940) decided that the question of upgrading the College to MBBS and that of coeducation should be considered as two separate issues. The boards finally agreed that Vellore could apply to the Madras University for affiliation for MBBS. They were informed that a Commission would be sent by the University to inspect the facilities and recommend whether the course could be started. Mrs. Peabody and the Board in New York were finding ways to raise finances as extremely difficult and Aunt Ida and Miss Dodd were keen to join her and others to provide an impetus to fundraising. Travel during the War was difficult and their furlough was indefinitely postponed.

The University Commission finally came in January 1941. It was an all male commission with many of the doyens of medical education in India, including Dr. Lakshmanaswamy Mudaliar, who would soon be appointed the Vice-chancellor of the Madras University as members. The Commission was impressed with the facilities on both the campuses, but their real concern was whether the College would be able to find adequate Indian faculty as salaries that were at best a fifth of what the Government would pay. The few Indians on the staff then, like Drs. Liza Chacko and Ebenezer Thomas, categorically assured the Commission that this was not an issue. As far as the pre-clinical subjects were concerned, Dr. Dorothy M Jefferson had completed her MS in Physiology and Dr. Liza Chacko had joined the Department of Anatomy and an extension to the Department was being built. The final report of the Commission recommending affiliation was submitted to the University who informed Vellore in May, five months after the inspection. They were granted permission to admit 25 women students for the preclinical course for two years subject to a large number of conditions, especially with regard to students progressing to the clinical years. Expansion of the Hospital and College buildings, additional equipment particularly for the laboratories, additional clinical facilities for male patients and recruitment of qualified faculty were absolutely essential before recognition to the clinical years could be considered on a temporary basis. Another university commission of inspection was scheduled two years thence to give final approval for the preclinical courses and to approve the clinical programme.

Aunt Ida and Miss Dodd left for the USA shortly after the inspection because she felt that where she was needed most was at the financial campaign. While they were in USA campaigning to raise funds for the College, Miss Dodd passed away after a brief illness. She was 82 years old and had spent three decades of her life supporting Aunt Ida in the pursuit of her vision. Her unsung contributions to Vellore were enormous. She was the Bursar and then Registrar of the School from the beginning, using the limited funds available with great responsibility. When necessary, her personal funds were generously used to meet urgent needs at the School. She supported at least six medical students in their course and innumerable projects at Vellore were quietly completed by her when available funds ran out. An example of this is the Clock Tower at the Hospital entrance, Miss Dodd contributed the clock and quietly provided most of the money for the Tower through the citizens of Vellore! To Aunt Ida, she was a close companion and friend, sharing her dreams and working shoulder to shoulder with her and her death left her with a sense of loneliness greater than when her mother left her in USA at the age of thirteen to return to India.

The first class of 25 girls was admitted to the MBBS course in July 1942. Aunt Ida was thousands of miles away, awaiting permission from the British Government to return to India and the appropriate visa. She had to wait till 1945 and the end of the War for this to happen. In the interim, she was part of a major drive to raise funds for the Medical College. She also was in the midst of discussions on admitting men into the College they had built for women to help the women of India. At Vellore, the faculty was convinced that co- operation with the NCCI and the CMAI was essential if additional faculty for the MBBS course were to be found from missionaries already in India. The Council had no doubt that what was needed was a coeducational college. However, the Board in New York, led by Mrs. Olson, the Chair and Mrs. Peabody, the Chief Fundraiser, were equally clear that for decades they had worked for a women's college and they would not allow it to be hijacked by men. Aunt Ida was caught in this chaos. This discussion continued and it was another five years before men were admitted as students.

Conclusion

Aunt Ida initially saw her continuing mission as training Indian girls to look after Indian women and children. As time progressed, priorities changed and the mission took on a broader meaning. The success of Dr. Ida S Scudder was that God gave her the wisdom to see priorities as they developed and respond to them. Her example has enabled the Institution to continue this important tradition.

The enterprising colleagues of Aunt Ida during this transition were Dr. Jessie Findlay, the Vice–principal who, as Acting Principal, guided the Institution through the difficult period of transition, and Dr. Chone Oliver, the Secretary of the CMAI who challenged the faculty and council to address the question of coeducation realistically. A crucial figure was Gertrude Dodd, Aunt Ida's constant companion who provided much of the funds for the College from her personal resources and was her confidant and adviser.

Aunt Ida's dream to train Indian women to look after their sisters and children, which started with the training of compounders with the help of Mrs. Gnanambal, the School of

Nursing in 1909, and the Missionary Medical School for women in 1918, culminated in the MBBS training programme in 1942.

The strength of the team that she had built up is shown by the fact that while she was away in America for four long years, Dr. Jessie Findlay, a Canadian missionary, supported by the Council in India, could go ahead and make the dream a reality by actually training girls for the MBBS and obtaining University recognition for the Institution.

Chapter 6

The Christian Medical College Vellore is Established 1942 – 1954

Dr. Jessie Findlay, Dr. Robert Cochrane, Dr. Hilda Lazarus

"July the first, 1942 was a Red Letter Day in our life as a College when the first MBBS Class was selected and 25 women students were admitted."

The opening sentence of the Acting Principal, Dr. Jessie Findlay's Annual Report to the Council in August 1943 started with the admission of 25 women for the MBBS programme. Yes, it was a landmark achievement but only a beginning. The provisional affiliation by the University of Madras was only for two years. There would be another inspection in two years to decide about continuing affiliation for the pre–clinical programme and for permission to start clinical training. Aunt Ida and Miss Dodd were in America, trying to raise funds for the College, a difficult task with America entering the Second World War in 1942. Miss Dodd passed away after an illness and Aunt Ida was stuck in the USA by travel restrictions due to the

Second World War. The debate whether the College should only be for women or it should be coeducational was still not settled. However, the faculty and the Council in India were clear that what they were aiming to build was the best medical college in India.

It was a good beginning, but there was a long journey before the College would be established and flourish. Recruiting an appropriate faculty and building the infrastructure for the College, including a 600– bed General Hospital to replace the Women and Children's Hospital were the urgent priorities. A General Hospital with at least 600 beds and Departments of Surgery, Medicine, Paediatrics, Obstetrics and Gynaecology, Ear, Nose and Throat, and Dermatology catering to men, women and children was essential for training and University recognition for the MBBS. It would be a formidable task to convert the Women and Children's Hospital staffed entirely by women doctors to a first rate General Hospital. Aunt Ida was 72 years of age and the key to success would be the response of the leadership inheriting the vision and mantle from her.

Inheritors of the Mantle

Aunt Ida was in the fifth decade of her devoted service to India. Her inspired leadership had fired the enthusiasm of a team of women missionaries dedicated to women's health to join her at Vellore and teach in the Missionary Medical School. In the staff list for 1942, she is shown as Principal (on furlough). In fact, she was held up in USA where she had gone soon after the inspection by the University Commission to raise funds. She would return to Vellore only in 1945 towards the close of the War. She unfortunately did not possess any university recognisable teaching qualification to be the Principal of an MBBS College. Aunt Ida and the Council had invited Dr. Hilda Lazarus to come and take over as Principal of Vellore in 1936. Dr. Lazarus, who was at the pinnacle of her distinguished medical service to India, was the Director General of the All India Women's Medical Service and had just been appointed the Principal of the new women's medical college in Delhi, the Lady Hardinge Medical College. In the middle of many problems facing the country, including the Second World War, she felt she should complete her service to India before she came to Vellore. The invitation was kept open. Who were the inheritors of Aunt Ida's mantle from 1942?

Dr. Jessie Findlay had been at Vellore with Aunt Ida since 1920. Appointed Vice–Principal in 1922, she was the Acting Principal during Aunt Ida's fundraising activities in the USA at the time of the first MBBS students were admitted. She was Aunt Ida's trusted colleague who gave leadership to the new college till 1944, but she did not have university recognisable qualifications. Dr. Robert G Cochrane, a distinguished Physician and Leprologist, in charge of the Leprosy Sanatorium at Chengelpet, was the Chair of the Vellore Council from 1942 to 1944. He had all the academic qualifications necessary for recognition by the University and agreed to relocate to Vellore, initially for two years as Principal and Professor of Medicine from 1944. Dr. Findlay welcomed this and decided she was too old to consider upgrading her medical degrees to allow her to be on the faculty. She handed over responsibilities to Dr. Cochrane and quietly returned to her Mission Hospital to continue her srvice as an outstanding surgeon for the next five years. As Acting Principal, teacher and Chief of the Department of Surgery, she earned the respect of all she served at Vellore –

patients, students and staff – for hers was a ministry of service. Her quarter century of service to Vellore from 1920 to 1944 was a major factor that helped Aunt Ida lay the strong foundations of the College. It was fitting that she led the College into the MBBS years.

Dr. Cochrane, while still in the Council, had requested Prof. CG Pandit, a distinguished Indian medical educationist, to inspect and give a detailed report on the strategy to develop the College. This blueprint guided the Institution in its early years. As Principal from 1944 to 1947, he was the architect of the new Memorandum of Association that was adopted by Council in 1947. Dr. Lazarus joined as Principal in 1947 as she felt she had completed her responsibilities to the Government of India. Dr. Cochrane was appointed to the newly created post of Director and served for a short while and in 1948 returned to his responsibilities as a Leprologist at Chengelpet. Dr. Hilda Lazarus was appointed as Principal and Director, posts she continued to hold till 1954 when she handed over the post of Principal to Dr. P Kutumbiah and Director to Dr. John S Carman. The development of the Christian Medical College during the formative years 1942 to 1954 was in the hands of Dr. Jessie Findlay, Dr. Robert Cochrane and Dr. Hilda Lazarus. Aunt Ida continued as Principal Emeritus, except for a brief period in 1946, when Dr. Cochrane was on furlough in UK when she was Acting Principal for about nine months. She presented her last Principal's report for 1945–46 in the August 1946 Council.

Recruiting faculty

The Principal's report to the Council in August 1943 clearly shows the lacunae in the faculty. In 1942, only three faculty had qualifications acceptable to the University: Dr. Liza Chacko MBBS, MSc in Anatomy, Dr. Dorothy Jefferson MD, MSc in Physiology and Dr. Ida B Scudder with her Diploma in Radiology from UK, although they lacked the necessary teaching experience. Four clinical departments were scheduled to be opened from January 1943 where "Professors" were listed (Surgery – Dr. Jessie Findlay; Medicine – Dr. KI Vaithilingam; Midwifery – Dr. Miriam Manual; Gynaecology – Dr. M Eapen). While they were all highly skilled clinicians, the highest medical qualification possessed by these four "Professors" was the MBBS or equivalent. The challenge to the inheritors of the mantle of Aunt Ida was to ensure an adequate faculty given the low salaries, poor infrastructure and the limited facilities in Vellore as a place to stay and bring up their families.

The Institution was also reeling from the resignation of Dr. Ebenezer Thomas, student of the first Diploma batch of 1918, given study leave to do the two–year short MB course in Madras and immediately on completion given further study leave, with full financial support by Miss Dodd, to obtain qualifications in the UK for Obstetrics and Gynaecology. She had just come back and joined the faculty in 1941 in this renowned institution.

After obtaining the MRCOG and FRCS qualifications, the University Commission during the Inspection in 1941 asked the Indians on the staff whether they would continue to work on the meagre salary offered. She and Dr. Liza Chacko in Anatomy, the only two Indians on the faculty at that time, emphatically assured the Commission that they would stay. However, soon thereafter, Dr. Ebenezer resigned and joined government service.

There were seven doctors working in the Hospital who were designated teachers for the university required departments to be started in January 1943. Apart from Dr. Gurupatham in Ophthalmology and Dr. Ida B in Radiology, none had postgraduate qualifications. Twelve years later in 1954, when Dr. Hilda Lazarus handed over the director's responsibilities to Dr. John S Carman, there were 22 teachers in the clinical departments with university recognised qualifications. The majority had been at Vellore for more than five years, and eleven of them were Indians including one Hindu. How did this remarkable change occur? Clearly, the efforts of the 'Inheritors of the Mantle' had been successful.

In 1942, at the start of the MBBS programme, Dr. Jessie Findlay was the Acting Principal helped by Dr. Carol Jameson, who had just returned after passing the FRCS examination in Canada, as Acting Vice Principal. They and the Council used four strategies to recruit faculty. The first was to request all missions working in India who were members of the Association to seriously consider transferring doctors with university recognisable qualifications to Vellore. Of course, this would be with the consent of the concerned doctors. It was also possible for those who did not have an appropriate qualification but were prepared to sit for an examination to be sent for training. This was essential to ensure the necessary clinical faculty in place at the review of university affiliation in two years.

This strategy paid off well and several missionaries already serving in India, inspired by Aunt Ida's vision, joined Vellore. The first among these as already mentioned was Dr. Robert Cochrane, a distinguished Leprologist as Professor of Medicine and Principal, in 1944. Two surgeons, Dr. John S Carman from the Baptist Mission Hospital Jammalamadugu in Andhra Pradesh and Dr. Norman S McPherson from the CMS Mission Hospital in Peshawar (now in Pakistan), joined CMCV in 1945. They were the pioneers who established CMCV as a referral centre for General Surgery and laid the foundation for the specialty departments of Urology and Plastic Surgery. Dr. McPherson had a British Postgraduate Degree that was recognised by the University. Dr. Carman took a year off to do the Canadian FRCP passing the examination at the same time as Dr. Jameson and then joined the faculty. Dr. Edward Gault and his wife Dr. Edna, Australian citizens, working in a Mission Hospital in Azamgarh in Uttar Pradesh also relocated to Vellore. Since Vellore already had two surgeons, Dr. Gault, a Surgeon, retrained as a Pathologist as he was expected to be the Head of the Department of Pathology, recognised as an area requiring urgent development to satisfy university requirements. Dr. Victor Rambo transferred from the Mission Hospital at Mungeli in Chhattisgarh to take charge of the Eye Hospital at Schell Campus. Dr. Donald Patterson in Radiodiagnosis and Dr. Herbert Gass in Dermatology were two more missionaries who relocated to Vellore in the mid 1940's, the former from China.

The second strategy was to request all missions and missionaries working in India to request their home offices to actively find qualified teachers for Vellore, recruit them as missionaries and send them out to Vellore. Five new faculty were thus recruited: Dr. Florence Nichols, Psychiatry; Dr. Ruth Myers, Microbiology; Dr. Paul Brand, Surgery; Dr. Gwenda Lewis, Anaesthesia; and Dr. Reeve H Betts, Surgery. Several others joined for short periods of service but did not complete at least five years or stay longer. After Independence, it became progressively more and more difficult to obtain permission for foreign nationals to serve in India as missionaries. A few more missionary faculty joined after 1954, but as those already serving went back home, the numbers gradually reduced and the last medical missionary at Vellore retired in 1993.

The next strategy was to try and recruit experienced Indian Christian doctors with university–recognisable degrees, who were willing to accept the low salaries at Vellore and prepared to relocate to what was then only a rather large village. Retirement from government service was at the age of 55 or 58 and such retirees could continue to serve as university-recognised teachers till they were 65 years of age. Dr. SC Devadatta, Professor of Chemistry in a Bombay college was recruited initially to the Physiology Department in 1946. As the role of Biochemistry increased in the curriculum, he developed the teaching department of Biochemistry in the College. Dr. Hilda Lazarus, a distinguished Obstetrician and educationist, first invited by Aunt Ida in 1938, joined Vellore in 1947, after completion of her commitments to Government service, as Professor of Obstetrics and Principal. She played a key role in the Institution as Principal and Director till 1954.

One of the most significant additions was Professor P Kutumbiah, who retired in 1948 from the Madras Medical College as Professor of Medicine and Principal. He was appointed as Professor and Head of the department of Medicine and was able to register students for postgraduate training leading to the degree MD in General Medicine from the Madras University. He took over as Principal when Dr. Hilda Lazarus retired in 1954 and served as Principal till 1957 and continued in the Institution till 1961. Professor Kutumbiah was an outstanding clinician and teacher who inspired many of his students to take up General Medicine as their specialty. Following him, Dr. JC David, Professor of Pharmacology, who retired as Principal of the Madras Medical College in 1954, joined as Professor of Pharmacology and Registrar of the College. He took over as Principal in 1957 and served till 1960.

The last, but not the least, in this group of Senior Indian Faculty who chose to hear and obey their call to Vellore was Dr. Jacob Chandy, an American Board certified Neurosurgeon in a faculty position in Chicago. He had trained with Dr. Wilder Penfield in Montreal and had joined Chicago a year earlier to develop Neurosurgery there. Dr. Lazarus invited him to come to Vellore plainly telling him that Vellore did not have anything to offer other than a position in the Department of General Surgery and the freedom to develop if he could find the means. Dr. Chandy's mentor Dr. Paul Harrison, an American missionary with whom he had worked earlier in Arabia, found some funds to buy essential equipment for Neurosurgery. Soon after arrival, he was called to see a patient with headache admitted under Professor Kutumbiah and diagnosed a brain tumour. With limited facilities, he operated successfully on that patient. This was the first neurosurgical operation in India, and Vellore never looked back. Dr. Chandy and the Neurological Sciences Department he started along with Dr. Baldev Singh, a Neurologist, achieved national recognition and initiated postgraduate training in Neurology and Neurosurgery. This first speciality department in India is still recognised as one of the best and has a distinguished record of training many of the Neurosurgeons who started academic departments in India. Dr. Chandy, with his many talents, served as acting treasurer, Medical Superintendent of the Hospital and Principal of the College till he retired in 1971. He was awarded the *Padma Bhushan* by the Government of India, recognising his sterling services to the country through Vellore.

The fourth and last strategy for strengthening the faculty was to recruit young Indian medical graduates and train them to get the required postgraduate qualifications for appointment on the faculty. This had already started in a small way with the students of the Licentiate programme. Ebenezer Thomas (class of 1918) Kamala Israel (1919) and Miriam Manuel (1926) were on the staff of Vellore in 1942. Ebenezer Thomas, the first Indian student to be given study leave and financial support, unfortunately left Vellore shortly after she obtained postgraduate qualifications from UK. However, Kamala Israel (Professor KI Vaithilingam) and Professor Miriam Manuel were faithful to their calling and gave a lifetime of service and more to their *Alma Mater*. The faculty, especially the expatriates tried to identify students who had the potential to join the faculty and encourage them to stay on in Vellore and offer a lifetime of sacrificial service. Four hundred and forty four students were trained to be MBBS doctors at Vellore, starting from the Class of 1942 to the Class of 1954. Thirty–eight of them joined the staff after completion of a postgraduate degree. Twenty–two of them stayed on and gave a lifetime of service to Vellore.

Anna Thomas from class of 1942, the first batch for MBBS, spent her entire life developing the Schell Hospital into a good Ophthalmology centre. Known for her sarcastic tongue, she was an excellent Ophthalmologist as well as a poet. Susan Benjamin (née Chacko) also of 1942, was an excellent teacher of Physiology. Rose Chacko from the Class of 1943 pioneered the Department of Psychiatry along with Dr. Florence Nichols and developed a unique system of in- patient care. Aleyamma Bhakthaviziam (née MP Aleyamma) was the best outgoing student of the Class of 1946 and the first winner of the Mariavyakulam David Medal in 1951 when she graduated. She chose Pathology as her specialty and made significant contributions to the development of the department. She married Dr. Bhaktaviziam of the Department of Dermatology. Another distinguished member of the faculty was Dr. Mary Verghese, who soon after graduation met with an accident and became paraplegic. She transformed this disability to a triumph by developing the specialty of Rehabilitation Medicine at Vellore. This was the first such department in India and a pioneering venture that helped to transform the lives of many paralysed patients. It has now become one of the premiere rehabilitation facilities in India. The Class of 1946 also contributed Dr. Sojibai Samson, who was part of the team who developed the Community Health Department which gave the distinction of being a community based Medical College to the Institution. Rachel Mathai (nee Eapen) a distinguished Dermatologist, who also served a seven– year term as the Medical Superintendent and her husband KV Mathai, the first neurosurgeon trained by Dr. Jacob Chandy, who also served as Associate Director during one of the most critical periods of the Institution, were the contributions of the Class of 1947, the first time men students were admitted to the College. CK Job also from the Class of 1947 was a pioneer in leprosy pathology and worked closely with Dr. Gault to develop the Department of Pathology. Jacob Abraham from the Class of 1949 was the second Neurosurgeon to be trained by Dr. Jacob Chandy for Vellore. He also served as the Medical Superintendent for a seven–year term and did considerable research on convulsive disorders and stroke in the community. P Zachariah who developed the Department of

Physiology after obtaining his D Phil from Oxford was the other contribution of the Class of 1949.

1950 contributed several members to the faculty. Abraham Verghese joined Rose Chacko to develop the Department of Psychiatry. Chinnoy JG Chacko was another member of the team that developed an outstanding Department of Pathology. Stanley John followed in the footsteps of Dr. Reev Betts to take the Department of Cardiothoracic Surgery to great heights. He was awarded the *Padma Shri* by the Government of India for his clinical contributions. Paul M Stephen in addition to being a distinguished Pharmacologist was the Official Choir Director and Organist of the College for many years. His baritone was distinctive. Grace Koshy placed Bacteriology at Vellore on the national map and helmed one of the best departments in the country. George Cherian from the same batch worked with Dr. Vaithilingam to develop Cardiology. Mary Sylvia Walter (nee Sonnell) worked along with P Zachariah in Physiology. Adolf Walter (1951) was a distinguished diagnostic Pathologist, but he is better known in the Vellore community for his brilliant Violin solos. Mary Jacob, who obtained her Doctorate in Anatomy from Oxford and spent her lifetime developing the Department of Anatomy also belongs to the Class of 1951. Joe O Devadatta, a skilled General Surgeon and brilliant teacher and Israel P Sukumar, a pioneer in Cardiology, who unfortunately died while in–service, were from the Class of 1952. Ramani Pulimood (nee Thomas) from 1953 and Saro Devanandan (née Vedamanickam) in 1954 complete the list of alumni recruited during this period. Although they were all identified by 1954, many acquired postgraduate qualifications and joined the faculty much later. They formed the backbone for the development of the Institution initiated by their mentors, the pioneers under the leadership of Drs. Jessie Findlay, Robert Cochrane and Hilda Lazarus.

There were several graduates of other medical colleges who joined Vellore as House Surgeons during this period, obtained postgraduate qualifications and joined the faculty and gave long service. They were P Koshy (1945) in Medicine, HS Bhatt (1946) Surgery, KG Koshy (1947) Community Medicine, Roy Ebenezer (1947) Ophthalmology, Daniel Isaac (1949) Medical Superintendent and in 1951 Arnold Desmond (ENT), AJ Selvapandian (Surgery, who then developed Orthopaedics along with Paul Brand), C Bhaktaviziam (Dermatology) and V Benjamin (Medicine and then Community Medicine). They brought a variety of diverse backgrounds and experiences, which contributed to the rich ethos of the Institution. Dr. Bhatt was the only non-Christian in this group but he identified with the ethos of the Institution completely. He was considered by many of his colleagues and students as more Christ-like in his commitment to the Institution and devotion to surgical work than many a Christian.

This group of professionals, all of whom excelled in their chosen areas of specialisation, ensured adequate faculty for the MBBS programme. As they grew in their profession, they started appropriate postgraduate programmes which brought the Christian Medical College to the forefront of medical education in the country. The excellence of the clinical care offered at Vellore and the commitment to Christ of the faculty ensured that all patients were treated as individuals with the love of Christ dictating all that they received.

Coeducation and MBBS

The closing sentence of Aunt Ida's Annual Report to the Council in August 1937 reads:

"We face the New Year with a calm assurance that if we follow closely, God will lead us into greater things for God keeps His Promises."

Vellore had just got the news that students could no longer be admitted to the Diploma programme and if the School was to continue, it had to upgrade to the MBBS course affiliated to the Madras University. There was also a serious financial crisis and a 10% salary cut implemented to overcome this, which was hurting all the staff, especially the lower paid. It would be four long years before students could be admitted to the MBBS in July 1942. Complicated negotiations with the boards in USA and UK as well as the Christian Medical Association (CMAI) in India were necessary. It is worthwhile to quote Minute Cl 411:1–1939 of the January 1939 meeting of the Council to give a flavour of these discussions and negotiations:

411. Co-operation with the Christian Medical Association of India in Christian medical education.

The Secretary read related correspondence with Mrs. HW Peabody and the Christian Medical Association and reported the results of conferences at Madras, December 10th, 1938 and Tambaram, December 28th, 1938.

Resolved that the recommendations of the Executive as presented to the Council be adopted and forwarded to the

Governing Board for their approval, after which it be sent as an overture to the Christian Medical Association of India.

"As a basis for consideration and motion by the Council, the Executive Committee recommend the following:

A. *That the Council reconsider the action of February 1938, and now declare its readiness to enter upon negotiations with the Christian Medical Association of India to found at Vellore a College which, with the existing Women's Medical College, Vellore, will form a coordinated institution for medical education of men and women.*

B. *That the general scheme of organisation be as follows :*

1. *That the Women's Medical College, Vellore, form a part of the larger institution; but for legal and financial reasons, it shall retain its own existing constitution.*

2. *That the Christian Medical Association of India set up a coordinated organisation for holding and controlling such funds and property as it may acquire.*

3. *That the existing Women's Medical College, Vellore, and the CMAI College when realised will be, for teaching and administrative purposes, one institution; and that as such it obtains recognition from the University of Madras.*

4. *`That there shall be:*

A Governing Council in India.

A President, who shall with the Council direct all the work of the Institution.

A teaching faculty composed of men and women professors.

A Dean of Men and a Dean of Women.

A Research Department.

One or more Hospitals.

A Nurses' Training School.

5. *That the combined Budget shall be made annually by the Council and be subject to approval by each coordinated body.*

6. *That co-operation as a coordinated institution begin as soon as agreement in principle is reached with the CMAI regarding the above scheme or some modification thereof, but that until co-operation actually begins, the Women's Medical College, Vellore, continue to operate independently and pursue the efforts to raise the existing School at Vellore to the MBBS Grade."*

All members of the Council who voted, voted in favour of these resolutions, two members abstained from voting.

No new students were admitted to the Women's Medical College at Vellore from 1938. By 1942, only the final–year students of the last batch admitted in 1937 to the five–year diploma programme remained and the faculty realised that unless students were admitted at least by July 1942 the affiliation of the College as a teaching Institution was likely to be lost. The critical factors apart from the concurrence of the boards were to bring up infrastructure by building and equipping a general hospital and laboratories essential for the College, such as pathology, microbiology and biochemistry, recruiting faculty and finding the funds necessary for operation. The strategy for recruiting faculty proved eminently successful and by 1941, the faculty felt confident to request the University to send a Commission to inspect the College to recommend affiliation to the University. The Commission inspected the College in January 1941 and recommended temporary affiliation for admitting pre–clinical students, to be reviewed after two years. The first batch of 25 girls was admitted to the MBBS programme in July 1942. The critical question left to be decided was whether CMCV should only be a Women's Medical College or should it be coeducational?

From the time the Christian Medical Association of India, with the leadership of Dr. Chone Oliver as Secretary, suggested in 1936 that Vellore should be the place where an All India Medical College admitting both men and women should be located there were two strong points of view. A group primarily in America, led by Mrs. Olson, the Treasurer of the Board and Mrs. Henry Peabody, a close personal friend of Aunt Ida who was responsible for raising most of the funds collected for Vellore, was clear that their inspiration was Aunt Ida's original vision to train Indian women to look after their sisters and their children. They were very clear that Vellore, Aunt Ida and all her supporters should stay faithful to her original vision and should only train women for the MBBS degree. The Board in New York supported this point of view. In contrast, the faculty and the Council at Vellore were equally clear that they were called to train both men and women and that was the only way to achieve excellence. At this time, the faculty were entirely missionary ladies and they were also the majority on the Council. The Board, the Faculty and the Council were all clear that they were following Aunt Ida's vision and her decision on this matter was crucial for the last word to be said.

Aunt Ida's first response when the idea of coeducation at Vellore was suggested was 'Over my dead body'! However, when the difficulties of developing a teaching hospital where men and women would of necessity have to be treated was coupled with her belief in the pursuit of excellence, she began to question her first reaction. The faculty at Vellore lead by Ida B, her niece, were equally clear that what they were called to develop should be the best Medical College in the country. When doctors from mission hospitals in India, many of whom were men, started relocating to Vellore, the consensus among the faculty for coeducation became stronger. The Council, almost all from mission hospitals, could see the need for trained men and women doctors. Aunt Ida was torn between the two choices. Should she remain true to her original vision or was God calling her to a new vision to develop the best Medical College in India training both women and men?

Soon after the inspection by the University Commission in 1941, Aunt Ida and Miss Dodd left for America to raise funds for the College. Ida B kept pressure on her Aunt to decide in favour of coeducation and finally Aunt Ida wrote to the Board in favour of co-operation with the CMAI to make a Christian Medical College for Women and Men in Vellore. The Board voted in favour of co- operation with CMAI to develop a coeducational college in December 1942. The resolution was carefully worded to permanently safeguard Vellore's commitment to women's medical education, by stating that at least 25 women students must be admitted each year! However, only women were admitted for MBBS in 1942, and it would be five long years before men were admitted in 1947. It is interesting that two words co-operation and co-ordination were used almost interchangeably to describe working with the CMAI to develop two colleges, one the existing one for women and the other an all India men's college. The Council Minutes record long discussion on how they were to be developed. Should there be two campuses or one, two hospitals or one? By 1945, these discussions petered out, wards for men were built on the Hospital Campus at Thottapalayam and quietly the first batch of ten men students were admitted in 1947 without much fanfare and with minimal additional facilities. Although there were no heated discussions in the Council or the boards at that time, this firmly established Christian Medical College Vellore as a coeducational institution. The sad repercussion of this change was that Mrs. Peabody and Mrs. Olson, two of the staunchest supporters of Aunt Ida and the College for almost three decades and who were responsible for raising most of the funds for the College, resigned from the Board in America in 1945 to record their serious protest at this dilution of Aunt Ida's vision. They could not accept that the vision given to Aunt Ida could change with circumstances and God dictated otherwise.

The role of Dr. Chone Oliver, a missionary doctor who spent almost three decades working in tribal India and two decades as Secretary of the Christian Medical Association of India, in persuading Aunt Ida and the Council to accept co–education as the better option was critical. The Council in Cl 738: 8–1946 acknowledged her contributions:

"738: Dr. BC Oliver. Resolved: That we place on record the appreciation of the Council of the Women's Missionary College, Vellore of the great service Dr. Oliver has contributed towards medical education in the past 20 years. If it had not been for Dr. Oliver's vision, ideals and persistence in the early days when few were convinced of the importance of a Christian Medical College,

there would not have been an all–India Christian Medical College today. Dr. Oliver's faith, courage and loyalty to her Master are a great inspiration to us, and this Council wishes further to assure her of their affection and prayers at this time."

This resolution followed Cl 737: 8–1946, which was a tribute by the Council to Aunt Ida as she officially retired from the College and became Principal Emeritus on August 16, 1946. The juxtaposition of the two resolutions highlights the importance of Dr. Oliver's contributions to medical education in India and especially to Vellore.

She retired from her five decades of work in India and went home to Canada soon thereafter. Sadly, she passed away almost immediately. The Council's Obituary recognising her role is quoted below [Cl 792: 8–1947]:

"In recording our deep appreciation of the life and work of Dr. Chone Oliver who passed away in Fort William, Canada, in May, we are moved to thank God on every remembrance of her – her years of medical missionary service at Indore, Dhar and Neemuch, her pioneer work among the Bhils at Banswara, her work as the first secretary of the Christian Medical Association, her founding of the Nurses' Auxiliary of the Association and her championship of the Christian Medical College Scheme. From 1902 to 1929, she served the Lord as a missionary doctor and from 1929 to 1946 as Secretary of the Christian Medical Association. After prayerful and very careful investigations of Ludhiana, Allahabad, Nagpur, Miraj and Vellore as to the most suitable place for a Christian Medical College for India, it was through her strong convictions, zeal and Christian love and hope that she was able to prevail on and win the consent and support of the founder of this College, our beloved Dr. Scudder, and the

Council and Board of the Missionary Medical School for Women, Vellore, to amalgamate with the Christian Medical College for India. Dr. Chone Oliver – one who always seemed so full of hope and cheer, she knew that there was nothing impossible with God and she went forth with a cheerful disposition, travelling far and wide over the breadth and length of India, often in a crowded third–class compartment. She was not over–blessed with robust health, and though in and out of hospitals as a patient, she still carried on her work to the very last in spite of pain and weakness. What she touched, she dignified and that dignity rested on sure foundations in her character. A firm faith in God and a constancy in prayer made her believe in great ends and also made her humble and human in her push for these ends. Her tact and her charm in human relations have ever endeared her to us. Those in mission hospitals will never forget her stalwart championship, her friendliness, her charm and her insight into their difficulties. She lived and worked for the Master who claimed her for His own."

Medical Students

When the 25 ladies of the first MBBS class were admitted, only the final year diploma students admitted in 1937 were still in the College. These girls graduated that year and the first batch of MBBS carried the Jasmine Chain to honour them. In many ways, life in the hostels was unchanged. 1942 was in the middle of the Second World War and life was full of deprivations and limitations. This touched the students little, except when the government requisitioned the women's hostel to house the police department being relocated from Madras. However, the Chief of Police was touched by the beauty of the Bagayam Campus and decided that the police did not deserve to be there!

Dr. Jessie Findlay, the Acting Principal and Dr. Ida B, the Acting Vice-principal heaved sighs of relief but still had to contend with all the other problems of the War years. The students of the St. Christopher Training College in Chennai were shifted to the campus and shared the hostel and other facilities with the Vellore girls.

Approximately, twenty-five women students were admitted each year till 1946. Ten men students were admitted in 1947 although the University had given permission for admitting twenty-five. The College restricted the number of men students till 1953 when 25 women and 25 men students were admitted. The residential facilities for men students were very limited with some buildings originally meant for servants, residences being modified for them with a thatched roof dining hall. Aunt Ida was very concerned about the facilities for men students and all the money gifted to her for her 80th Birthday in 1950 was put towards the hostel. The beautiful and very comfortable hostel on the other side of the road from the College and the women's hostel was completed and occupied in 1952. This was the last building that was built by Mr. Rottschaefer before he retired from Vellore. His was a remarkable career being responsible for all construction at the Hospital and College from its inception. Money would be paid in advance to him on the basis of an estimate and when construction was over it would be measured independently and payment settled at government Public Works Department rates plus 5%. The quality of the construction was excellent as he built for the centuries and cost was less than that of any contractor.

The traditions developed by the students of the Medical School for Women were carried on and built upon by the

MBBS students. This was symbolised by the last Diploma batch presenting a Gold Medal to the College President of 1942 as a Badge of Office, which is still handed over by each president to the successor. The ceremonious Jasmine Chain procession where the graduating class is escorted to the Hall by the final-year students shouldering a Jasmine Chain interwoven with leaves is a symbol of the unique traditions that have developed for and by the CMCV students. Unfortunately, some of these traditions like the semi-formal Sunday lunches in the hostels attended by staff and their families have weakened and are no longer practised. The Foster Child programme started in the early fifties where one or two students from each class is adopted by a faculty family resident on campus and offered privileges of their home is still active and is one of the major forms of bonding with students.

Life in the College

Grants from the British Government were a major source of support to the College, apart from the money collected by the Boards in USA and UK. In 1943, the College was informed that there would be no further grants and the College would have to be truly self-supporting. As the faculty and Council discussed how to live with this reality, three principles for the future Governance of Vellore evolved:

1. *The College should be owned by Indian Churches.*

2. *The College Administration should be Indian.*

3. *The College should generate funds in India for its work.*

The invitation to Dr. Hilda Lazarus to come to Vellore to be Aunt Ida's successor can be considered the first move in this strategy. Although she was first invited in 1936 her sense of responsibility to the Country and to the Government she served meant that she assumed this responsibility only by 1947. From the start of the College till the Constitution of the Vellore Christian Medical College Association was adopted in 1947 the Chief executive officer of the Institution was the Principal, a post held by Aunt Ida till 1942 when she was designated as Emeritus Principal. Dr. Jessie Findlay was the acting Principal in 1942 and she continued till1944 when Dr. Cochrane joined Vellore. Significant decisions during her time were the co–operation with the Madras Medical College for teaching pre– clinical and clinical students till the expansion of the Hospital was functional and the discussion on admitting men students for MBBS. Dr. KI Vaithilingam was given study leave to do Postgraduate training in Medicine at Madras Medical College.

Dr. Robert Cochrane was a distinguished Leprologist working at the Chengelpet Sanatorium near Madras. He was a member of the Vellore Council representing the Church of Scotland Missionary Society and was the Chair of the Council from 1942 to July 1944. His academic qualifications were acceptable to the University. He was offered and accepted to join the faculty for a two year period or till the end of the war whichever was longer and joined as Associate Professor of Medicine and Principal from August 1944 [Cl 512; 7–1942]. Dr. Findlay handed over the responsibility of the College to Dr. Cochrane. She went back to her Mission for a further 5 years as a Surgeon before retiring from India.

Dr. Cochrane was the architect of the Memorandum of Association, Constitution and Bye Laws that were adopted from 1947 [Cl 7–1942: 595 and Cl 8–45: 663]. The CG Pandit review of the Institution was commissioned by Dr. Cochrane when he was the Chairman of the Council and it provided the blue print for development. The method of selection of undergraduate students was formalised with a theory examination, an in-depth interview at Vellore for more than two days with objective tests and subjective assessment. The selection strategy was developed with the help of Dr. Frank Lake, who served on the staff for two years. The report to the Council in August 1946 showed that 178 students applied for the test from whom 80 were called to Vellore for assessment. Seventy of them came and 25 girls were chosen and admitted after evaluation, including one Hindu and one Muslim. It was also decided that upto 80% of the seats in the Medical College would be for candidates sent from the contributing missions. This was in response to a request from the Government in Madras that 80% of admissions should be from the Madras Presidency. The College replied that since most of the supporting churches were in the Madras Presidency, it is likely that most of the students were from there. This was the first of many attempts that continued till the next century by the State Government to have a decisive say in the running of the College. None of these attempts were successful even before the Constitution of India gave a fundamental right to religious and linguistic minorities to establish and administer educational institutions of their choice.

A major crisis was the resignation of Mrs. Peabody and Mrs. Olson from the American Board following the approval of the Institution becoming coeducational. The contributions of Mrs. Peabody, who first visited Vellore and spent a day with Aunt Ida in 1913 and was inspired by her vision for the development of women's medical education at Vellore and specifically the Campus at Bagayam are not often remembered a century later.

She and Mrs. Olson, who was the Treasurer of the Board in New York, were responsible for raising and sending all the funds for the construction of the Hospital at Thottapalayam and College buildings at Bagayam. This partnership between Aunt Ida and Mrs. Peabody played a critical role in the development of the College. She had visited Vellore in 1938 at the 20th Anniversary of the College and had been honoured by the College and the Council for her exceptional services to Vellore. She believed firmly that the decision to become coeducational was a betrayal of Aunt Ida's original vision and she would no longer be associated with the work at Vellore. Unfortunately, she could not accept that this was not a betrayal but a God–guided expansion of Aunt Ida's vision and her pursuit of excellence for His glory in the service of India. The Institution owes the memory of Mrs. Peabody a debt of gratitude and it is worth quoting the tribute Council paid her in CL 666:8–45:

"Mrs. HW Peabody: As a Council we desire to give expression to our deep appreciation of the monumental work of Mrs. Henry W Peabody in the establishing of the Missionary Medical College for Women, Vellore. Up to 1945, the building progress was due to her efforts more than to any other one individual. In her relation to Vellore, we are reminded of the story, 'The Last of the Giants', written by one who visited mission institutions in this part of India. Mrs. Peabody came to India as a missionary in her youth, and her children were born in India. She was later active in many time–consuming projects in North America and was known from coast to coast for her valiant fight for Prohibition. She was largely responsible for the establishment or re–birth of the seven women's Christian colleges in Japan, China, and India. The Women's Christian College at Madras and the Isabella Thoburn College at Lucknow, along with the Missionary

Medical College for Women, Vellore, are institutions for the Christian training of India's womenhood that largely benefited by her inspiring ardour. During the campaign for funds in North America for the seven colleges, she considered her day wasted did she not at least make three public addresses. She and her family are equally well known for their Christian labours in the Philippine Islands. Even now, with more than fourscore years, she is still much sought for as an inspiring devotional leader. There are few such women in any one generation. We at Vellore desire to express our heartfelt gratitude to her for making this Institution possible, and do assure her of our unfailing resolve to share with her, her ideal which is, we believe, the presentation of Christ as Saviour to the young people of the world."

Dr. Cochrane took a short furlough in 1946 and Aunt Ida acted as Principal during this six–month period, her last official activity at the College. She officially retired from Vellore after many farewell functions on August 19, 1946. The note in her diary that day 'Left Vellore. Oh it was so hard to say goodbye' expresses not only her feelings but that of the whole Institution who also did not want to say farewell. She continued as the esteemed Principal Emeritus, spending the summer months at Hill Top, her home in Kodaikanal and the cooler months of the year at Vellore. She was the inspiration of all who came in contact with her and continued to be an inspiration to many and the guardian of our traditions.

The new Constitution outlined in [CL 663:8-45] was crafted by a Committee of three, Dr. Cochrane, Rev. CR Wieranga, the Council Secretary and Rev. JC McGilvray, the Treasurer. The Institution owes a burden of debt to the formulators of this Constitution because it laid the basis for the governance of CMCV. The fundamental objective of the India registered association in whom the ownership of the Institution would vest was clearly spelt out as education and research. The draft of the Constitution was approved in August 1946 [Cl 725:8–1946] and the Constitution was formally accepted in the March 1947 meeting [Cl 781:3–1947] and the Objects of the Association as stated in the Memorandum of Association states:

"The objects for which the Association is set up are:

1. The establishment, maintenance and development of a Christian Medical College and its associated hospitals where women and men may receive an education of the highest grade in the art and science of Medicine and of Nursing, to equip them, in the spirit of Christ, for the relief of suffering and the promotion of health, hereinafter called the primary object. In the Medical College provision shall be made for approximately equal number of men and women."

[Cl 725:8–1946, Appendix VI page 36 August 1946 and Cl 781:3] 1947).

The Board that essentially owned the College till then composed of Churches in America with missionary bodies working in India. The membership in the Association was opened up as shown in Article 1 below:

"Any Christian Church, Association, Society or Missionary Body jointly approved by the Association and Board, which for the purpose of co-operating "in the support of "the College contributes or engages to contribute Rs. 6,000 per annum (or its equivalent) or such sum as may, from time to time, be agreed upon by the Association at its several meetings in consultation

with the Board, shall be "a subscriber to and a member of "the Association."

The fundamental intent of this Constitution was to ultimately change the ownership of the College to an Indian Association, composed of the Indian operations of the missionary societies who formed the Board in New York and to open the membership to Indian Churches. This intent was clearly stated in the report that accompanied the Constitution as follows:

"The Committee recommends to the Council that it give careful consideration to the following statement of policy: "While it is desirable that the Institution should not lose its present international character, whenever a vacancy occurs, first consideration should be given to the appointment of a suitable candidate of Indian domicile. Further, especially in making appointments to junior posts, the College should seek: in every way to build its own leadership."

This new Constitution began the Institution's journey to becoming an Indian organisation. The second major change was that the post of a Director was defined as the Chief Executive Officer of the Institution, the sole channel of communication between the Council and the College. The administrative structure was formalised and duties of all Administrative Officers were defined, giving overall authority to the Director. The formal transfer of ownership to the Association to India was completed at the next major revision of the Constitution in 1955.

The Council in 1947 was made up of less than twenty organisations, each represented by up to two individuals, seven co-opted members and one representative each from the

Senatus and the Medical Board formed after the revision of the Constitution. At the March 1947 meeting, 42 names are listed with five Indians, one representing the Arcot Co-ordination Committee, three co-opted and one from the Senatus. In August 1947, the number of members had increased to 53 but the number of Indians remained as five, including Dr. Lazarus, the newly appointed Principal. However, the intent of the Association to indigenise was clear in the new Constitution. The membership of the Council showed significant changes by August 1954. There were 24 members of the Association including two Indian churches represented by 70 individuals of whom 17, including Dr. Lazarus, the Principal and Sir Samuel Ranganathan, the Chair of the Council, were Indian.

Hilda Lazarus was appointed as Principal in August 1947 and Robert Cochrane moved to the newly created post of Director. Dr. Cochrane decided to move back to Chengalpet by March 1948 to continue his research and treatment of leprosy. The rural outreach centre in Kavanur (Kilvaithankuppam), about 20 kilometres west of Katpadi on the Gudiyattam road became a reality. This was initiated by Dr. Cochrane as part of his leprosy outreach work. Dr. Cochrane in his final report to the Council said:

"Let us therefore continue with no thought of race, but with one purpose only–that India, our beloved India, shall through our contribution as a Christian Medical College advance in scientific knowledge and spiritual attainment towards that position in the Councils of the Nations which we believe she is destined to take.

May our work help to bring to this land a unity of purpose and a spiritual stature which will enable her to assume her place as a natural leader of the East."

This prophetic wish has been more than fulfilled.

Dr. Lazarus was appointed as Principal and Director in March 1948. [CI 837:3–1948]. Soon thereafter, she went on a promotional visit to UK and USA for fundraising. Carol Jameson was the Acting Director and Principal for about six months during this time and Aunt Ida was requested to be in residence at Vellore as Emeritus Principal, Dr. Gault was appointed as Vice–principal and Dr. Macpherson as Medical Superintendent. The six years Dr. Lazarus was in charge were years of growth and stabilisation of the MBBS programme.

A detailed method for selection of undergraduate students for the MBBS course, aimed at evaluating a candidate's 'Suitability for training at CMCV' was established in 1947. This included an all India entrance examination to grade the academic and non-academic knowledge of the students. The All India Entrance Examination was designed to assess not only their academic knowledge but also their general ability and importantly Christian knowledge. This was essential since students applied from all parts of India and academic standards varied widely. Approximately, double the number of candidates as there were seats were invited for a detailed evaluation at Vellore in which their general ability was assessed by a series of objective tests and their commitment and desire to do medicine, evaluated by in–depth interviews by senior faculty.

This system of selection with periodic fine–tuning continued until the second decade of the twenty–first century when it had to be changed due to changes in national laws controlling admission to the myriad medical colleges that had sprung up after India gained Independence. A full discussion of this issue is beyond the scope of this book. Tension developed between the medical and nursing faculty and a special committee was appointed to look into this problem.

The rules and regulations regarding staff was codified and approved by the council [Cl 915;8–1948]. A committee consisting of Drs. PV Benjamin, JS Carman and RH Betts was given the responsibility to plan and implement upgrading all the Departments in the College thus stimulating their development [Cl 918:8–1948]. It was decided that in the interest of the Institution, study leave could be given to confirmed faculty even before completing five years of service, a decision that led to upgrading the skills of faculty and also providing them an opportunitytoearnsomethingextradependingonthefellowships they obtained [Cl 919:8–1949]. The sabbatical programme was started by permitting faculty who had completed five years of service to take three months leave on full pay [Cl920:8–1948]. The Malakara Orthodox Syrian Church was admitted as the first Indian Church to the Association [Cl 924:8–1948]. In view of the leprosy work started by Dr. Cochrane, the relationship of the Institution with the Leprosy Mission was clarified and research work in Karigiri as an independent but related institution was started. [Cl926;8–1948].

One of the significant decisions of 1948 was the payment of House Rent Allowance at 20% of Basic pay to all the staff [Cl 942:31949]. Major General Wilson Haffenden who retired from the Colonial Government was appointed as the first full– time General Superintendent [Cl 978:3–1949]. Although he retired after just over a year, his contributions to an efficient administration were so good that the post has been in effect since then. Another significant appointment in 1949 was of Miss Anna Jacob, a Vellore nursing graduate who had obtained postgraduate qualifications as the first Indian Nursing Superintendent.

The optimum number of medical students to be admitted was set at 50 each year after a careful evaluation [Cl1002:8–1949]. An interesting observation was that fans could be provided to faculty resident in rented housing with the provision that they would not have to dismantle and return them to stores at the beginning of winter season! [Cl 1005:8–1949]. An internal telephone system was established costing Rs 10,000/–, an indication of the recognition of optimal communication as essential for development. It was also recognised that building more private rooms for paying patients was essential for improving the finances of the Institution [Cl 1009:8–1949].

1950 was the Golden Jubilee of Aunt Ida having started her work in Vellore and this great achievement was celebrated appropriately with many grand and gala events at Vellore. One of the highlights of the year was that the Madras University, thanks to the efforts of the Vice–chancellor, Dr. Lakshmanaswamy Mudaliar, a great friend of the Institution, ensured that the letter of Permanent Accreditation of the Vellore MBBS course was delivered to Aunt Ida at the major meeting celebrating the jubilee, as a fitting tribute to her. Rev. Sanjeevi Savarirayan, who had obtained experience in hospital administration, applied for the post of General Superintendent as suggested to him by Dr. Jacob Chandy and he was appointed to the post full–time [Cl 1062a:2–1950]. Faculty would be given permission to attend

International Scientific conferences with full pay, but they would have to find the money for travel from other sources [CI 1100:2–1950]. There was a strange decision that the General Superintendent should be the executive head of the Hospital [CI 1042:2–1950]. This decision was found impractical and rescinded in 1952 [CI 1547:8–1952]. Dr. P Kutumbiah was appointed as Principal from 24 February 1950 [CI 1141:8–1950]. The State Government insisted that unless 50% of the seats for MBBS were kept for admitting non–Christian students, the capitation grant for the maintenance of the College would be stopped. This condition was unacceptable to the College and since then it has been run as an unaided college without government grants [C I1161: 8–1950]. An attempt was made to prepare two five–year plans for the development of the College, but nothing concrete was achieved.

Dr. JC David was appointed as Professor of Pharmacology and Registrar of the College from March First 1951. The policy to encourage departments and units to develop their Special Funds to be used for development and continuing educational activities like attention at conferences was approved [CI 1270:2– 1951]. Many building projects were approved including a Neurology block [CI 1305:2–1951]. The policy to take external loans for development that would pay for itself in a short time period was approved [CI 1331:8– 1951]. A new X–ray machine was purchased at the cost of Rs. 40,000/–. This is the first recorded capital expenditure for equipment and was the forerunner of equipments being a major item of expenditure as medicine embraced technology to a greater extent [CI 1342:8–1951]. Significant grants were received during the year from a variety of sources including Rs.1.5 Lakhs for the development of Thoracic Surgery and $25,000 for Neurosurgery [CI 1343:8–1951].

The optimal number of medical students to be admitted each year was decided to be 50 [Cl 1552: 8–1952]. The State Government again demanded that 50% of the seats in the MBBS programme should be given to non–Christian candidates if the grant–in–aid was to be continued. The Council again rejected this demand [Cl 1556:8–1952]. Dr. Brand and Dr. Carman presented the draft of a proposal for a special Rural Medical Scheme. The Council approved further studies and a grant from the Wellcome Trust in London to study this further [Cl 1668:2–1953]. The first training programme in Clinical Pathology for technicians was started admitting 15 students [Cl 1678:2–1953].

Dr. Hilda Lazarus, who had served the Institution with distinction since 1947, requested that she should be relieved as soon as possible.The Council agreed to relieve her from March 1954 and appointed Dr. John S Carman, Professor of Surgery as acting Director till the search committee could present their recommendations to the Council [Cl 1619:8–1953]. The University formally recognised the Institution for the MD postgraduate programmes in Pathology and Obstetrics and Gynaecology [Cl 1726:21954]. Since Dr. Kutumbiah joined, CMCV students had been recognised for training for MD in Medicine but since only one student passed in the seven years till 1954, there were no applicants for the course! The final draft of the Rural Medical Scheme was approved and this led to the Rural Hospital on the Bagayam Campus.

Building and Infrastructure

The tradition at Vellore was that new buildings are always necessary to provide the infrastructure for the ever expanding medical work. The pressure on building became very acute since the different university commissions pointed out the need for meeting the minimum standards of infrastructure set by the University. From 1921, CMCV was fortunate that one of the missionaries of the American Arcot Mission, the Rev. Rottschaefer was an excellent architect and engineer. He took on the responsibility of managing all the building work that was necessary. The buildings were built to last centuries and we owe Rev. Rottschaefer for much of the buildings on the Campus. The minute of appreciation by the Council spells out the Institution's debt of gratitude.

"It is with very great regret that the Council has learnt of "the resignation of Dr. B Rottschaefer from our building programme, and we would like to place on record our deep debt of gratitude for his long and splendid service as Builder of the Vellore Medical College and Hospital. From the very inception of the Missionary Medical School for Women in this place almost thirty years ago, it has been one of the fortunate circumstances attending this Institution that a person like Dr. Rottschaefer was available to build the innumerable buildings. There is not a stone or a brick in the structures of these magnificent edifices that does not bear witness to his efficiency and the integrity of his character. For sheer durability and dependability, we know of no series of buildings to compare with Vellore Medical College, for they are a translation into stone of the spirit and ideals of the founders of this place, and they will stand as a monument of his skill and will ever live in the hearts of the hundreds of women and men who have studied in and visited them. Not only as Builder has Dr. Rottschaefer made his devoted contribution to the College, but he has given his services at all times freely and in manifold ways. All his wise guidance and advice in legal and complicated matters has saved the Institution thousands of rupees and has always been at the disposal of the Council and its Executive Committee. We look forward to the continued participation and cooperation of Dr. Rottschaefer in such deliberations in the future as in the past, for he has proved an invaluable colleague who has helped to preserve the standards and build up the traditions of the College, our venture of faith in the service of the Master." [Cl 769:3–1947]

Many of these buildings still stand as witness to the honesty and professional ability of Rev. Rottschaefer and his commitment to the institution.

Finance

The inheritors of Aunt Ida's mantle commendably ensured the viability of the institution for the education of young women and men, training them for the relief of suffering in the Spirit of Christ as the primary purpose, recruiting faculty and developing appropriate infrastructure. One of the critical concerns was ensuring the finance for staff salaries and technological development. Sixty percent of the income of the institution was provided by grants from the Boards in 1942– 43, and the first–year MBBS students were admitted. Aunt Ida's reputation as a caring Christian doctor and a superb Obstetrician and Gynaecologist became the reputation of the institution for all–round excellence in providing healthcare as skilled faculty were recruited. The direct result of this was a significant growth in the number of patients, increasing the income from Rs. 30,386/– in 1938–39 to Rs. 9,61,888/– in 1953–54. The expenses also increased, including salaries, capital expenditure for improving the technology for patient care and physical infrastructure, including accommodation for the faculty. Given the limitations of Vellore, which was only a large village, suitable accommodation for staff was a high priority. Council decided that even amounts designated for endowments should be used for building accommodation as they realised the essential nature of providing facilities for staff. The Council also realised that as more Indian staff were recruited, the question of income from private practice, consultations and university examinations would become an issue and with foresight passed a rule to take care of such contingencies:

"Cl 866:3–1948. Policy regarding the receipt of examination fees, etc., by members of staff. It was Resolved : that payments received by members of the staff for private or outside consultations, examining fees, lecture honoraria, etc., shall, in accordance with tradition and the practice generally prevailing in mission hospitals, be regarded as part of the income of the Christian Medical College and payable into its funds. Actual expenses incurred are of course payable out of such fees. This ruling cannot be made applicable to members of staff engaged before the present date, but it is hoped that it will meet with the concurrence of all concerned."

Salaries were modest and apart from accommodation provided by the Institution, there were few financial privileges. As the numbers of locally recruited staff increased, one of the privileges available to them was to go for specialty training to enhance their skills. Where it was necessary to acquire a university recognised degree for teaching designation, study leave was granted to other Indian Institutions, but all staff were encouraged to go abroad for training. In addition to enhancing skills, this helped to develop valuable contacts with their mentors which helped in long–term development of specialties.

It was also possible to save some money from the scholarship towards a nest egg to start savings.

The Council considered the question of savings or pension at the time of retirement. The supporting missions had their own arrangements for their missionaries. The only person not covered by her mission, Dr. Degenring, who had spent almost 20 years with Aunt Ida was provided a pension by a special Council resolution. There were several discussions in the Council about providing a pension especially for the very low salaried Indian support staff. The deficit budgets each year having to be topped up by grants from the boards left no balance to consider futuristic decisions on pension plans. In fact, one of the local auditors, who had worked with the Income Tax submission for faculty for many decades, said in the early 1970's that he knew that God approved of the work at Vellore because the Income Tax paid by all retired faculty increased exponentially after they retired from CMC!

Conclusion

The decision by the Madras Government to abolish the Licentiate training programme in Medicine and the decision of Aunt Ida, the faculty at the School and the Council supported by the Board to start the MBBS training and then to make a coeducational institution resulted in amazing growth and development at Vellore leading to the establishment of the Christian Medical College at Vellore with a remarkably good faculty and a reputation for excellence. Aunt Ida's mantle was inherited by Jessie Findlay, Robert Cochrane and the first Indian Principal Hilda Lazarus. When Dr. Lazarus retired in 1954, the College had grown to 50 medical students admitted each year, postgraduate programmes in Medicine, Surgery and Obstetrics, a strong College of Nursing and begun training technicians to work in Hospital Laboratories and in Radiology. Aunt Ida was no longer involved in the day–to–day running of the College but was the source of inspiration to all.

Chapter 7

The Carman Years: Development, Specialties and Postgraduate Education, 1954 – 1967

Dr. Hilda Lazarus handed over a College with an established MBBS programme admitting both women and men and a six–hundred bed Hospital, recognised as one of the best in India, to Dr. John S Carman on the First of March 1954. In addition to training students for the MBBS programme, the College was recognised by the Madras University for the MD degree in Obstetrics and Gynaecology, Medicine and the MS degree in General Surgery. There were two units in Obstetrics and Gynaecology, three each in Medicine and Surgery and a good Paediatric Department. The original Mary Taber Schell Hospital was a full–fledged Ophthalmology Hospital with Dr. Victor Rambo, a pioneer in community Ophthalmology and eye camps. A community health outreach and research programme was in the process of being established by the Department of Preventive and Social Medicine under the leadership of Drs LeRoy Allen and KG Koshy. The College Campus outside the town on the Hill site at Bagayam, with excellent facilities and accommodation for students and limited accommodation for faculty and staff, was developing into a good residential campus.

Two important policy documents were adopted by the Council at their meeting in February 1954. A report by a committee headed by Dr. Paul Brand recommended that a village–based hospital, to train medical students in rural medicine should be started, if possible in a village

Within a mile or two of the college, failing which it could be started in the mango orchard which formed part of the college campus. This idea was accepted by the council, and, with financial support from the Wellcome Trust and the Nuffield Foundation, the rural hospital at Bagayam near the junction bus stand was started by Dr. LeRoy Allen and KG Koshy. They adopted the Kaniambadi Rural Development block to the South of the College Campus as the field practice area [Cl 1719:2–54]. The other recommendation was by a Committee headed by Dr. MacPherson, Professor of Surgery who had spent many years in mission hospitals in India. The Council accepted [Cl 1727:2–54] that all staff to be accepted as permanent faculty should undergo three months of Bible training. The memorandum outlining this was accepted by the Council and referred to the Director to bring back recommendations for implementation. In the next Council meeting, it was suggested that the course run by the YWCA of India in Ooty each summer could be used for this purpose but it did not become a regular part of faculty appointment.

Constitution

A major revision of the Constitution and Bye laws of the Association, drafted by a Committee chaired by Dr. Jacob

Chandy, was accepted by the Council in August 1955 [CI 1854:8–1955]. The purpose behind this revision of the Constitution was to conform to the realities of post–independence India. The membership of the Association, the owner of the Institution, was limited to churches or Christian bodies that were Indian. The ownership had vested with the Board in New York till this Constitutional revision. Provision was made in Article VII Membership of the Council, the body tasked with governance of the Institution, for appropriate representation of the missions and churches from outside India, who in fact were the owners till then. This change was a major policy change and the then Council Secretary in Appendix II to the minutes stated as follows:

"Among these newfound rights of men are the right to freedom and the right of self–determination. Nothing else is treasured so highly. They are products of Christian teaching, and democratic indoctrination. From the standpoint of Christian training and Christian service, it is a matter of utmost importance that these be kept firmly Christian in character and aligned to Christian goals.

It follows that all Christian work in India, as in other lands, ought to become firmly rooted in India itself. Its sense of possession ought to reside in the Christian Church and Christian organisations of the land; only then will it thrive in the new atmosphere. This awareness calls for a change in the Constitution of the Association and Council of the Christian Medical College. The Constitution as proposed will acknowledge the College as belonging to the Christian people of India; it will continue to recognise co–operation with the Ecumenical Church through its various parts the world over by a Council representing contributing bodies in proportion to the amount of aid received."

The Council Minutes have a detailed analysis comparing the 1946 Constitution with the new 1955 Constitution. The Memorandum of Association in four parts defines the name of the Association in the first paragraph as "The Christian Medical College Vellore Association". Paragraph 2 adds "promotion of health" to the list of Objectives. Paragraph 3 defines the Powers of the Association and Paragraph 4 restrains the Association from getting any financial assistance that will interfere with its primary objective of "imparting education to young women and men in the Spirit of Christ". The Constitution and its Bye laws are the basis of the smooth functioning of the Institution and its harmonious relationship with the Association and its Council. The Constitution emphasises that the Christian Character of the Institution be maintained to ensure that the ethos of the Institution continues to grow as envisaged by the founders.

Comparing the 1955 Constitution with the present (2021) Constitution helps to appreciate the foresight of the framers of the document in 1955. Ten of the sixteen articles in the Constitution of 1955 have not required any amendment till 2021. The details of the amendments to the other six articles reflect significant changes in the life of the Institution. Article I, Membership of the Association that owns the Institution, was expanded and clarified, but continued to be restricted only to Indian churches and Christian bodies. Starting with only two Indian churches and organisations in 1954, it grew rapidly and by 1957 had twelve Indian churches and Christian organisations as members. Many of these were Indian missions and churches that were initially founded by overseas churches by their mission activities.

In Article II, a small Nominations Committee defined in the Bye laws replaced the Executive Committee (EC) for nominating Officers of the Association and membership of the EC, thus ensuring that the Executive Committee does not become a self–perpetuating body! An important tradition that has been established is that while the term of the Council Secretary may overlap the term of the Director, a new secretary is usually nominated by the Director and elected by the Council. This recognises the reality that the Council Secretary is the key liaison between the Director and the Council and its Executive Committee and has to have the absolute confidence of the Director. Article VII, Membership in the Council has been expanded to give appropriate representation to sister institutions and the considerably increased faculty and staff. Article VIII now includes the provision for a Chair pro–term in the absence of the Chair and Vice–chair. In Article IX, the powers and duties of the Council original Clause 1.d is now divided into clause d and e for greater clarity. In Article XII defining the duties of the Director, provision has been made for Associate and Deputy Directors to help the Director, as administrative work increased with the size and complexity of the Institution. There were no major changes in any of the other Articles, sixty–five years after they were accepted.

Planning for the future

In his report to the Council in the first year as Director, Dr. Carman spelled out his priorities and plans for the future development of the Institution:

"On the other hand, it seems to me more realistic for us to recognise the earning capacity of this Hospital and to strengthen

the work that is done in such a way that we will have a more normal relationship between private and general ward patient accommodation and care than we have had during the period of trying to meet University requirements. The demand is great for specialty services. The waiting list is often long for private room accommodation."

It was realised that the future depended on raising finances for day–to–day running of the Institution by charging realistic fees to those who could afford to pay for clinical services and wanted private room accommodation, not on expectations of grants from overseas missions. The Institution was offering clinical services of high quality, valued by patients and the Director's priority was to increase the quantum and quality of these specialised services. He was keen to modify salary scales to offer remuneration for clinical staff which, while not competing with government or other private institutions in India, would still attract Indian healthcare professionals who were keen to serve and train in the spirit of Christ. The policy was to serve an adequate number of private patients to ensure funds for the care of those who required free or subsidised care. It was recognised that increasing the reputation of the Institution would require enhancing the scientific productivity of the faculty, leading to academic excellence based on clinical excellence. Inviting specialists as visiting consultants to help develop new clinical services was one strategy that was spelt out. Further development of postgraduate training with new specialties and their involvement in research projects was prioritised by the faculty. Modification of salary scales and the provision of better retirement benefits was identified priorities. However, the Director recognised that capital expenditure would still require external grants and it would be his responsibility to secure such grants for development.

An interesting vignette is Dr. Carman, in his first Director's report to the Council, thanking Dr. Lazarus for preparing him over time to take over the responsibility as Director. This cordial system of training and handing over responsibility from one director to the next, established by the Institution's third Director, Dr. Hilda Lazarus to the fourth, Dr. John Carman is a unique tradition that continues till today and now covers the handing over of responsibilities by all Administrative Officers. The successful operation of this strategy is dependent on the successor being identified at least three months prior to the completion of term of the incumbent so that they can work together for a smooth and seamless change.

Realising that more Indian faculty would be appointed and that missionaries are likely to decrease in number, an important policy decision was enunciated. Missionary societies provided for extended home leave for a year, usually after a period of five years of continuous service in India. This time was used not only to visit family and assist in raising funds but crucially for acquiring new skills to enhance services at Vellore. It was a sign of great forethought when the Council approved a sabbatical leave for Indian faculty after five years of continuous service [CI 1684:2–1954]. The period of six months on full pay or a year on half pay for each period of five years of service to a maximum of 15 years, with seniority and other privileges protected was unique to CMCV until very recently. An approved programme of skill enhancement was the basis of granting this leave. Obtaining an appropriate placement and necessary funds for a sabbatical was the responsibility of the faculty with guidance from the Institution. The sabbatical could not be used to do private practice in India but could be used to work in a mission hospital. Most faculty were able to arrange programmes, which in addition to skill enhancement would also provide good emoluments and the savings during this period were usually significant in providing financial security to staff on a salary much lower than their peers in India. The skills acquired and contacts established during sabbaticals have helped in the development of several specialities at Vellore.

An important financial policy was enunciated in the February 1954 Council Meeting [Cl 1701 and 1702: 2–1954]. Building eight guest rooms for patients and their attendants, and an additional floor over the fourth wing of the nurses hostel to shift staff nurses who were occupying rooms in the private wards were identified as 'self– liquidating' projects where income generated by the facility would be sufficient to settle the debt incurred for building and would, after the debt was cleared, generate income for the Institution. Council accepted that borrowing from external sources such as banks would be justifiable under those circumstances and an external loan of Rupees Sixty Thousand was approved. This policy decision has helped the Institution thereafter in planning capital and development projects judiciously.

Other important decisions in 1955 included attempts at payment of retirement benefits and pension (not immediately possible due to financial constraints), starting a Cost Accounting section to ensure that realistic fees were charged to patients, clarifying rules regarding sponsored candidates for MBBS selection and regularising appointments under special funds. Government of India sponsored the attendance of Prof.

Liza Chacko, the Head of the Department of Anatomy at an international conference, and this was commended by Council as a recognition for her and the Institution to be emulated by other faculty.

The Faculty

Dr. Carman in his Director's Report to the Council in 1954 unequivocally stated his policy for the future development of faculty: "In the scientific world, and this is no less true of the medical and the associated sciences, an institution or any one of its staff becomes known and is judged by being 'productive or non-productive'. The products should be scientific papers of high grade as well as young people trained to add to the body of knowledge in the various sciences. We are coming to a time when our own staff, new or old, will have to be judged according to the criteria of their productivity as well as in other standards. I am glad to say that quite a number of our staff have attained eminence along these lines. The rest of us must come up to standard." The focus on academic productivity by the faculty ensured that the Institution stayed in the forefront of academic medicine and excellent patient care as it grew over the years.

The Institution was already recognised by the University to train postgraduate students in Medicine, Surgery, and Obstetrics and Gynaecology. One student had obtained her MD in General Medicine by then. Several attempted the MD examination after fulfilling the university required training, but none were successful in the examination until 1960 when George Cherian of the batch of 1950 passed the examination on the first attempt. Dr. HS Bhatt was the first to obtain MS in General Surgery. He joined Surgery Unit 1 headed by Dr. Carman. The Medicine and Surgery departments were divided into three units, each with areas of specialisation. Medicine Unit 1 under Prof. P Kutumbiah chose Haematology and Gastroenterology as their areas of specialisation. This focus was sharpened by the arrival of Dr. Selwyn J Baker, supported by the Church Missionary Society in 1955. He had trained under Prof. JV Dacie at the Royal Postgraduate Medical School at Hammersmith in the UK and started Research on Nutritional Anaemia. He quickly realised that the majority of nutritional anaemias seen at Vellore were megaloblastic anaemias and showed that in non–pregnant adults both Vitamin B12 and Folic Acid deficiency occurred in association with a malabsorption syndrome. The Wellcome Trust provided funds to support this work and also to establish a ten–bed metabolic ward with a well equipped laboratory in the basement below the ward. Dr. Selwyn started the tradition of employing fresh graduates with a service obligation to the Institution as Research Fellows to work on specific projects which were not necessarily clinical. Dr. KI Vaithilingam returned about the same time after working for a year with Helen Taussig in New York and was in charge of Medicine Unit 2, where she developed the specialty of Cardiology. Dr. Philip Koshy developed Nephrology as the special focus of Medicine Unit 3. He obtained the first artificial kidney in India, a Kolff Unit, through a donation by a patient.

An interesting anecdote. Dr. Koshy obtained the Kolff kidney by March of 1961 and went to Seattle for appropriate training. While he was still away, the patient who had donated the kidney deteriorated steadily and went into uraemic coma. His family were very upset and complained to Dr. Carman who sent a cable to Dr. Koshy in Seattle. Dr. Koshy replied by cable: 'Ask Mathan to dialyse the patient!' I was a house staff in

Medicine Unit 3 and Dr. Koshy had called me and Mohan Luke, a Biochemist he had employed, and asked us to be in charge of the dialysis machine and keep it safe. Dr. Carman called me and showed me the telegram and asked what I would do. It was clear he expected me to follow Dr. Koshy's order. I asked for a day's time and with Mohan Luke, studied the instruction that had come with the dialysis unit, successfully dialysed a stray dog and were confident that we could manage the machine. As per Dr. Carman's instructions, we then dialysed the patient successfully, the first use of the artificial kidney in India. The patient woke up from coma and talked to his family, but with the inexorable progression of renal failure lapsed back in coma in about 72 hours. We again dialysed him and he woke up. Three days later, when he again lapsed into coma, the family were content to let nature take its course. In my assessment, the Kolff kidney was excellent for dealing with acute renal failure when a couple of dialysis could be lifesaving, but not ideal for chronic maintenance dialysis. Of course, new technology took care of this but by then I had moved on to other interests!

Dr. John S Carman was in charge of Surgery Unit 1, assisted by Dr. HS Bhatt with Urology as their area of interest. Dr. Paul Brand, with his interest in rehabilitative surgery for leprosy patients, initiated the specialty of Orthopaedic Surgery in Surgery Unit 2, along with Dr. AJ Selvapandian. When the Orthopaedics Department was given a separate identity, Surgery Unit II continued as a general surgical unit with Dr. AS Fenn as the chief and developed an interest in paediatric surgery. Dr. NS MacPherson was in charge of Surgery Unit 3 and the special interest of this group was in Head and Neck Surgery and Plastic Surgery. The Department of Obstetrics and Gynaecology was divided as two units under Dr. Paranjothi and Dr. Miriam

Manuel. The Departments of Dermatology (Dr. Herbert Gass) was part of the Division of Medicine, while Ear Nose and Throat Surgery (Dr. Albert Patt), Neurological (Dr. Jacob Chandy) and Thoracic surgery (Dr. Reeve H Betts) as well as the Orthopaedics Department (Drs. Paul Brand, AJ Selvapandian, MV Daniel) were part of the Division of Surgery.

The identification of potential future faculty especially from among the students in the College, their nurture and further training was a major priority of the administration during this period, and the faculty actively worked for this. Several Indian doctors who were not Alumni, but who had obtained their postgraduate degree abroad were recruited as they returned to India. This was facilitated by a Scheme of 'Pool Officers' initiated by the Department of Science and Technology of the Government of India. This scheme encouraged Indian professionals to come home, guaranteeing a good salary from the government for two years or earlier till they were able to find a suitable permanent opening in India. The Department of Medicine was fortunate to have several excellent teachers under this scheme, Hari Vaishnava, Sarala Vaishnava, XJ Ankelesaria, FM Narielwala and SK Vaish. These excellent clinicians and teachers served on the faculty for two to ten years and provided a challenging academic atmosphere for the students. All of them moved on to senior faculty positions in other medical colleges in India. Their presence and academic excellence were a stimulus to those going through their undergraduate training at Vellore at that time and the Institution was able to recruit many of these students to the faculty. The Department of Surgery on the other hand recruited Christian graduates of government medical colleges and trained them for faculty positions. Outstanding examples of this are Dr. AS Fenn and Dr. LBM Joseph. The Department of Paediatrics was strengthened by Dr. Sheila Pereira and Dr. Malathy Jadhav, graduates and postgraduates from other colleges who identified totally with the ethos of Vellore. Dr. Benjamin Pulimood, a graduate of the Trivandrum Medical College joined Vellore as a House Surgeon in 1960, then went to the UK, obtained MRCP from Edinburgh and returned and joined the faculty in 1965. He served for nearly 30 years as Professor of Medicine and Head of Medicine Unit 1, Principal and Director. In 1961, Jacob John, also from the Trivandrum Medical College, joined as house staff in Paediatrics and then went to UK, did his MRCP and returned to Vellore in 1966 to develop the Virology Department.

Several graduates of Vellore were recruited after obtaining their postgraduate qualification through the Institution during this period. Many of them gave a lifetime of service. Sarojini Vedamanickam (Devavanandan) from the Class of 1954 served a lifetime in the Department of Anaesthesiology. Vimala Muthiah (Charles), a Gynaecologist worked till 1967 and resigned from service. The Class of 1955 gave the Institution several faculty most of whom gave many years or a lifetime of service. Minnie Thomas (Mathan) specialised in Gastrointestinal Pathology and Electronmicroscopy and was an internationally recognised expert in the field when she superannuated in 1997 as Professor of Gastrointestinal Pathology. Dora Hemalatha (Rao) also specialised in Pathology and served Vellore till 1977 along with her husband M Mohan Rao, a Urologist responsible for the first renal transplant in India in 1971. This was the beginning of the well– established renal transplant programme at Vellore, which by now has done over 1000 transplants in the last 50 years. Mani M Mani along with Dawson Theograj of the 1952 Batch, pioneered plastic surgery at Vellore but they both resigned in 1973, feeling that the academic powers at Vellore were not supportive of the development of this specialty. Marcus S Devanandan obtained his PhD in Physiology and served on the faculty till his superannuation as a Neurophysiologist. In August 1961 shortly after graduation, VI Mathan working as Junior House Surgeon in Medicine, was requested by Dr. Selwyn Baker to lead a Field Research team investigating an outbreak of Epidemic Tropical Sprue in and around Wandiwash about 80 km southeast of Vellore. He continued to work with Dr. Selwyn as he pursued MD in General Medicine, which he obtained in 1965. He then joined Medicine Unit 1 to continue research on diarrhoeal diseases. This research group was supported by substantial grants to Dr. Selwyn Baker from The Wellcome Trust, London. Dr. Selwyn Baker resigned from Vellore in 1975. Mathan developed a multidisciplinary team with expertise in Clinuical Gastroenterology, Epidemiology, Gastrointestinal Pathology, Biochemistry, Microbiology and Virology. The work of this multidisciplinary team on enteric infections was recognised as an 'Advanced Centre for Research on Enteric Diseases' by the Indian Council of Medical Research in 1990. A Clinical Department of Gastrointestinal Sciences was also developed out of this research unit in 1972 by Mathan and it has now grown into one of the leading centres in Gastroenterology in the country. Mathan, in addition, served as the Council Secretary from 1984 to 1991, the Medical Superintendent from 1988 to 1994 and then was selected as the Director of CMCV for three and a half years, till his superannuation in 1997.

Lily Thomas (John) from the Batch of 1956 was Professor of Medicine and Head of Medicine Unit 2 until her superannuation. Prakash Khandhuri gave a lifetime of service as a General Surgeon, developing Hepato–Pancreatico–Biliary Surgery at Vellore. He took over Surgery Unit 1 when Dr. LBM Joseph was appointed as the Director in 1976. Prakash was an outstanding surgeon and a passionate teacher who contributed significantly to Vellore's reputation as a centre of excellence. KE (Dicky) Mammen worked with AS Fenn to develop the Department of Paediatric Surgery. Dr. Thomas Sen Bhanu was an excellent surgeon in Oto–Rhino–Laryngology. Molly Kurien (Bhanu) followed JC David in the Department of Pharmacology and also developed a Clinical Pharmacology Service. 1957 contributed K Kuruvilla to the Department of Psychiatry and Annie Verghese (Sudarsanam) to Clinical Pathology. Her contributions to Blood Banking along with Bob Carman were noteworthy. Shanker Krishnaswamy from the 1958 Batch played a major role in developing and strengthening the Cardiology Department started by KI Vaithilingam after IP Sukumar (Class of 1953) and George Cherian (1950). Hemalatha Airon (Krishnaswamy) a stalwart in Pathology, and Alice Abraham (Kuruvilla) in Pharmacology were others from 1958 who gave a lifetime of service.

The 1959 and 60 batches were admitted, half to a premedical year (Physics, Chemistry and Biology) and the other half to the First year (Anatomy and Physiology) of the medical curriculum, due to changes in university regulations making the one year Pre–University the basic requirement for admission to the medical course after the University abolished the two–year Intermediate programme. BS Padankatti in Physical Medicine and Rehabilitation, Sushil M Chandi in Pathology, AM Cherian in General Medicine and Bhooshanam V Moses in General Surgery were recruited from these two years. Bhooshanam served as the Principal for seven years and established an excellent rapport with the students. Meshchak Kirubakaran of 1961 worked with Dr. P Koshy and KV Johnny to develop the

Department of Nephrology towards the first renal Transplant in India by M Mohan Rao (1955). Daleep Mukarji of the 1964 Batch developed the Rural Unit for Health and Social Action (RUHSA) starting from 1976 as a major community outreach programme of the Institution. He then went on to serve as the General Secretary of the Christian Medical Association of India (CMAI).

1964 was also the year Joyce Ponnaiya (MD Pathology), who served as Principal and Director, joined as a student. Serving as Director from 1997 to 2002 Joyce was responsible for successfully celebrating the Centenary of the Institution. Rajaratnam Abel, who followed Daleep Mukerjee at RUHSA, also belonged to the 1964 Batch. His leadership of this major project of the Institution established it as a major teaching and research unit in a truly rural area. Vinod Shah from 1964 Batch gave a major impetus to distance education at CMCV, especially for the staff of mission hospitals scattered in remote areas in rural India. Alka Ganesh, who was Professor of Medicine at Vellore and Ganesh Gopalakrishnan, who continued to develop Urology after Mohan Rao, belonged to 1965. The last year of this period, the Class of 1967 gave the Institution David Sadhu as Professor of Surgery and George Chandy, who became Professor of Gastroenterology and served as Director for a five-year period. The best outgoing student of the Class of 1967, Mammen Chandy developed the specialty of Haematology at Vellore and established the first bone marrow transplant programme in India at Vellore.

The efforts by Dr. Carman and colleagues to recruit faculty from among the graduates of Vellore succeeded beyond expectation. The recruitment was facilitated by a Faculty Cadre periodically determined by the Cadre Review Committee and approved by the Council. The selection of staff is a careful process involving the Heads of Departments and Units, the Administrative Officers and the Staff Selection Committee. The Cadre Review and Staff Selection Committees are two of the several standing committees of the Council which have faculty participation and have played a major role in the development of the Institution. By the end of the Carman Years, the selection of faculty primarily from among those who do their postgraduate degrees at Vellore had been well established. This has led to the faculty being primarily chosen from most who have done their undergraduate training and all with postgraduate training at Vellore. In reality, this ensures that the majority of the medical faculty are Christian with a sprinkling of outstanding non-Christians and that the traditions and culture of the Institution is maintained. The dangers of inbreeding have not yet manifested, probably because of the opportunity for a three-year study leave, again facilitated by the Study Leave Committee, soon after confirmation on the faculty and periodic sabbaticals ensuring that external influences leaven the faculty. The smooth and harmonious functioning of these committees, all of which are chaired by the Director and some of which have Council members also as members has been the lynchpin of participative management.

Standing committees of the Council

Over the years, the Institution developed a set of committees which ensure inputs from the faculty and external experts to guide the way forward. This system has been found to be one of the strengths of the Institution. Bye-law V of the Constitution and by-laws of the Association currently (2021) lists fourteen Standing Committees of the Council. The 1944 Constitution and by–laws do not list any committee other than the administrative committee. As the Institution grew in size and complexity these committees evolved to fulfil felt needs. These fourteen standing committees can be broadly classified as six committees that primarily deal with administration and the council, six that deal with academic matters and two that oversee sponsorship of students for admission by eligible members of the association. The Director is a member of all these committees and is the Chair or Convenor of all but one of them, the Staff Selection Committee is chaired by the Council Chairman. The composition of these committees, their powers and duties are spelt out in the by–laws and are hallowed by traditional practice over the years. All these committees have effective participation by the faculty, a tradition that started when the faculty were almost all overseas missionaries who also represented their missions in administrative responsibilities. As more Indian faculty were appointed, they naturally took on the responsibilities which were held by the missionary faculty they replaced, facilitating the smooth indigenisation of the Institution.

Committees that deal with Administration and the Council

The Administrative Committee: All the administrative officers serve along with currently five staff at the professorial level elected by the Council for two–year terms, constitute the Administrative Committee (AC). There are no external members in the AC. The AC is chaired by the Director and the General Superintendent is the Secretary. The primary responsibility of the AC is to approve all financial actions for later ratification by the Council and to assist the Director in the administration of the Institution. All Administrative Officers will bring any matter that requires a decision to the AC agenda with the prior approval of the Director. The agenda of the Executive and Council meetings is made from the resolutions of the Administrative Committee and reference to the Council minutes show that almost all of them have reference to the relevant AC minute number. Ordinarily, the AC meets once a week, currently on Thursday afternoon and the agenda is circulated to all members in advance. The representation of five professorial level staff in the AC ensures that staff participation in decision–making is effective.

The Planning Cell: All administrative officers and four other Council–appointed staff elected by the Council constitute the Planning Cell. This committee is responsible to advise the Council through the Director for the planned development of the Institution. It is interesting that, while on paper, the Planning Cell is an excellent idea for futuristic planning, several Directors have used the AC for planning and not used the Planning Cell. It is worth considering whether the Planning Cell plays a really constructive role or should quietly be dropped from the list.

The Finance Committee and the Building Committee have strong representation from external experts and are Technical Advisory bodies to guide the Administration. These committees have no staff representation other than Administrative Officers. Members of staff may be invited when matters relating to their departments are considered. The Chaplaincy Committee has representation from the hostels as well as the students and at least three pastors of local churches. The Nominations Committee consisting of the Director, the Council Secretary and three members elected by the Council is responsible to bring nominations for co–options to the Council, nominations for the offices of the Chair and Vice–chair, and the membership of the

Executive Committee and all other standing committees of the Council.

Committees dealing with academic and student affairs

The Cadre Review Committee: It is essential for excellence in academic matters to ensure the optimum cadre of faculty. The Cadre Review Committee ensures periodic analysis of sanctioned faculty strength and recommends appropriate revisions and necessary increases commensurate with developmental activity and workload in he College. It is against the sanctioned cadre that faculty are appointed after appropriate screening of credentials by the Screening Committee and review of their recommendations by the Staff Selection Committee chaired by the Chairman of the Council before presentation for approval by the Council. In the case of faculty appointments, such recommendations have also to be approved by the University who ensures that academic credentials are appropriate before formal appointment orders can be issued. While there is only one Staff Selection Committee cadre review and screening are done by different committees for each academic stream, Medical, Nursing and A llied Health streams.

Student Selection Committee: Separate student selection boards are constituted for each academic stream, Medical, Nursing and Allied Health Sciences. The selection boards are formed by all faculty and others involved in the selection process and they finalise the marks awarded to candidate students. The final selection is then done by the respective selection committees. The Director, Principal, Medical

Superintendent and Council Secretary are members of all selection committees, Medical, Nursing, and Allied Health Sciences. The Principal is the Chair for all selection committees except those for nursing students, which are chaired by the Dean, College of Nursing. Council elects one member annually to serve on these selection committees. The professors and heads of departments of all departments involved in particular streams of training are all members of the respective boards.

Screening Committee: The responsibility of the Screening Committees is to ensure that the academic credentials of all individuals are appropriate for selection or promotion by the Staff Selection Committee. Appointment or promotion is dependent on availability of vacancies in the sanctioned cadre of each department or unit. Ordinarily, individuals are appointed as junior lecturers after completion of postgraduate qualitification by the Principal against vacancies in the sanctioned cadre.

Staff Selection Committee: The final recommendation on the appointment or promotion of all Council–appointed staff is the responsibility of this Committee. The Chairman of Council, the Director, Principal and two members of the Executive Committee, who are not on the staff, form this committee. It is responsible for the final review and recommendation of all appointments and promotions to the Council for approval.

In the 1950s and 60s, there were many vacancies as listed earlier many of the students completing postgraduate degrees were immediately appointed. The process at that time was rather informal. I was informed by Dr. Vaithilingam, the Professor of Cardiology and Head of the Department of Medicine, who was one of my examiners, that I had passed the MD in General

Medicine in the evening of the day of the Practical and Oral examination in Chennai (Madras). I came back to Vellore by a night train and met the then Principal Dr. Jacob Chandy the next morning to inform him of the happy news and to request an immediate appointment as a Junior Lecturer. He suggested that I join Dr. P Koshy in Medicine Unit 3 but I requested that I should be posted in Medicine Unit 1 with Dr. Selwyn Baker. While there was vacant cadre in Medicine Unit 1, there was no budget provision for further appointments and I requested that I be posted as Junior Lecturer, Medicine, in The Wellcome Research Unit for which Selwyn was responsible. Since research funds were available and for the preceding four years, I had been informally involved in the Unit's field research activities, Dr. Chandy immediately agreed and I started working the day after my MD Practical examination. Of course, an appointment order was issued several months later when the results were announced and back–dated to April 15. A year later, I was promoted as Lecturer in Medicine after Screening Committee and Staff Selection Committee processes, Council concurrence and then the approval of the University! Since to most of us appointed at that time the timely receipt of salary was essential for day–to–day expenses, this informality was a great boon. Of course, things are much more formal now.

The Academic Committee: The drafters of the Constitution were very clear that the primary activity of the Institution was education. The responsibility of the Academic Committee was to "provide independent external expertise for the formulation and maintenance of educational standards and to ensure excellence, national impact and social relevance in the academic activities of the College, including research consistent with the mission and objectives of the Association". This Committee chaired by an eminent medical academician/scientist has twelve external members including the Secretaries of the Departments of Biotechnology and Health Research of the Government of India, nine eminent scientists/academicians, and six faculty from the Institution including the Principal, Director and Dean, College of Nursing.

Being a student – 1955 to 1966

Training undergraduate students was and continues to be the core of the Institution envisaged by the Founder. The first training course started by the Founder was for training Pharmacists (Compounders) primarily because a trained person was available to run the Course! As the Institution grew, many other courses evolved. It was realised

That excellence in clinical and public health service is the key to excellence in training in health sciences. A hundred and twenty years after Aunt Ida started her clinical work, the Institution offers over 50 different training programmes showcasing excellence in–service and outstanding education at the undergraduate and postgraduate levels in Allied Health, Nursing and Medical Sciences. Higher specialty training leading to the MCh or DM degrees after basic postgraduate courses were pioneered by the Institution in the early 1950s starting programmes in Neurosurgery and Cardiothoracic Surgery.

Life in the College now, the third decade of the twenty–first century, is very different from what it was in the 1950's, almost seventy years earlier. I was admitted as an undergraduate medical student in June 1955 and after graduation completed my MD in General Medicine and joined the faculty as a Junior Lecturer in Medicine in 1965, ten years later. I look back on those ten years through rose–tinted glasses, but will try and describe them as realistically as possible. The students admitted till 1947 were all women and in the early 1920's lived with Aunt Ida and Dr. Elizabeth Findlay almost as a family in a very small Institution struggling to establish itself in an alien environment in India. The total staff at the inception was less than twenty with just Aunt Ida and Jessie Findlay as the teachers. Three decades later, by the mid–fifties the Institution had grown with a total staff of about 600 of whom less than a hundred were faculty. The Hospital had only 600 beds with a very busy out–patient service as many patients had to be managed as out–patients due to limitation in beds. A large proportion of the patients had been referred to Vellore as a court of last resort or for getting specialised diagnostic tests. Patients could pay and obtain private consultation

A large number of students of their Intermediate College course, which has now been discontinued, would hope to get themselves to a medical college. To prepare for, they would have taken biology, physics and chemistry as their optional subject. Government colleges admitted on the basis of these marks at the University examination giving preference to socially and economically weaker students. This meant that the competition for the merit seat was fierce. Vellore gave preference to students who were sponsored by the churches that supported the Institution. These students gave a commitment to return and work in those hospitals for at least two years, in the hope that they would then commit to a longer period of service. While 90% of the seats were reserved for such students, 10% of the seats were available for meritorious students based on their performance in the entrance examination, which was at the time held by the Institution. This is now replaced by the National

Eligibility and Entrance Test (NEET), which is common for all institutions and has made life of students much easier. Based on the performance at the entrance exam as well as Church support, approximately double the number of seats (then it was 25 men, and 25 women) would be called for a detailed interview and test to assess their suitability to be trained at Vellore. This three–day interview was usually from Wednesday.

The names of those selected were announced on a Saturday afternoon and I went to the main post office in town to send a telegram home with the good news. When I came back, the candidate who shared my room in Men's Hostel had almost finished packing and I helped him carry his bags to the second gate to catch a bus and start his journey home. It was a quiet evening and a night of good sleep, waking in the morning to go for the first service at St John's Church in the Fort. After lunch, it was ensured that all the new students were in rooms on the A and B block ground floor and we all had rooms to ourselves as all the unselected candidates had left Vellore, we had a quiet and peaceful Sunday afternoon and all were encouraged by the seniors to attend the College Chapel for which very little persuasion was needed, as we were filled with gratitude to God for our selection.

Returning from the Chapel, we were surprised to see that the Men's Hostel was completely dark and ominously quiet! Those who went straight for dinner were routed via the Lily Pond and had to change before dinner! This ducking in the pond was the beginning of the formal process of welcoming us to the hostel! Classes started on Monday and the hostel welcome activities continued for a week till we were formally inducted members of the Men's Hostel Union (the Mansion of the Gods) at the

Fresher's Dinner the following Saturday night. Part of the ritual was that our classmates of the opposite sex were special guests of the men students for the evening. A few of us chose a guest but the majority were assigned a guest and I am afraid I cannot remember who was my guest!

Classes started in earnest on Monday morning with the lecture in Physiology by Dr. Dorothy Jefferson followed by an Anatomy lecture by Dr. DL Graham and then the introduction to the cadavers, half the class starting the dissection of the upper limb and the other half, the lower. We quickly realised that if we were to give full justice to our studies, our involvement in the extracurricular activities would have to be carefully planned. In the premedical college course, I was actively involved in the Basketball, Cricket and Tennis teams of my then college. I had to choose one of these in the Medical College, and I chose basketball as among the three I enjoyed it most. On retrospectroscopy, it was probably the wrong choice as I could not continue to play basketball as a junior and trainee doctor and certainly not as junior or senior faculty. The court was in the College Campus and even when we got a court made in the Hospital where was the time or the energy? Probably, tennis would have been a better choice. The details of undergraduate training are in Appendix 3 and are not repeated here.

Immediately after completion of Compulsory Rotating Internship, I joined in January 1961 as a House surgeon, as it was a requisite before I could register for the MD in general medicine programme. While doing a six month posting in Medicine Unit 3 with Dr. P Koshy, I realised I had a problem. In the first clinical year, Prof. JC David who was the Principal called me and offered me a good scholarship which was based on my excellent academic record and the fact that my parents were retired teachers in a Christian College with a low salary and no pension. This help was most welcome and reduced the financial burden on my parents. I was surprised one Saturday a few months into my internship when Mrs. Carman, the Acting Treasurer of the College called me and asked me to sign a legal document that I would serve wherever the College asked for a two–year period because of the scholarship given to me. Rather than start a fight, which I had no moral right to win but could have won on legal grounds that it was not informed to me prior to the grant and acceptance of the scholarship, I signed the bond realising that this meant I had to work for two years in an area of need as decided by the College and would have to defer my postgraduate studies by two years.

Six months into my Junior house job, as I was finishing my posting in Medicine in Unit 3 where I helped in establishing the artificial kidney programme, Dr. Selwyn Baker offered me a chance to lead a field team to investigate an epidemic of diarrhoea in Wandiwash and the villages surrounding that district headquarters town about 80 km south–east of Vellore. The field team consisted of myself, two interns doing their Community Medicine posting in rotation for six week periods, three technicians to run a field laboratory, a driver and field survey staff who would have to be recruited. We recruited two health inspectors who had retired from government service as they had field experience and would know how to deal with the village administration. The whole team was to stay in Wandiwash, the headquarters town (glorified village) of the Taluk (administrative sub–division of the District) of Wandiwash. It was a challenging opportunity to do something different and also offered a good salary which was most welcome as I had become engaged to be married to my classmate. I started this posting for a year on August First 1961 and agreed for a year of adventure. A major motivating factor was that the Administration agreed that this year would be set off against one of the two years of service obligation for the scholarship, but it turned out to be one of the best decisions of my life as it determined the direction of my entire professional career.

We would start our week in Wandiwash on Sunday evenings as we spent the weekend at Vellore. Around 5 AM, the field team would leave for the village we were surveying that day as all those villages were agricultural and the people would be off to the fields at sunrise. We would be back in our accommodation by 9 AM and after a quick breakfast run a clinic for patients with diarrhoea. After an afternoon siesta, the field work would again start by 4 o'clock and go on till eight at night. Saturday, we would return to Vellore after lunch, a two–hour drive. The field team had two internes from the community health posting to assist me, two or three fieldworkers who would do house to house surveys in the affected villages, two technicians for the laboratory where tests of intestinal absorption and basic haematology and microbiology tests were done under field conditions.

Six villages within fifteen kilometres of Wandiwash were selected for detailed survey and about 60 villages in that area were kept under surveillance to detect new outbreaks of diarrhoea. We collected a lot of information and established that at least a hundred thousand patients, mainly adults, were affected with diarrhoea which continued for weeks or months and in some cases for years. All available evidence, including that from the 1961 census, showed a high mortality in this region confirming our field data. All patients investigated both in the field and back at the metabolic ward in Vellore had intestinal malabsorption and developed signs of nutritional deficiency. We called this disease "Epidemic Tropical Sprue" after establishing that starting as an acute episode of diarrhoea, the majority of those affected continued to have symptoms for four weeks or more and manifested malabsorption of dietary nutrients in the first week of illness, leading to malnutrition. The field work started in August 1961 but the peak of the epidemic was over by October–November 1960 and we were unable to establish causality or find the aetiology.

This research project was funded by a special grant from the Wellcome Trust in London to Dr. Selwyn Baker. The Trust had earlier funded a ten–bed metabolic ward and a research laboratory for Selwyn's work on malabsorption syndromes and megaloblastic anaemias in the Tropics. After a year's work at Wandiwash, I relocated to Vellore and completed my house job by spending six months in the Casualty Department to fulfil the minimum requirements for admission to the MD programme. I continued to work with Dr. Selwyn to study the epidemic irrespective of what other responsibility I had. The University had sanctioned three seats for admission to the MD training programme each year. I was the only applicant in March 1963 as hardly anybody from Vellore had passed the MD examination of the Madras University for nearly ten years. Most students preferred to go to UK to do the MRCP (Edinburgh), which was recognised by the University for teaching purposes. CK Eapen in 1961 and VX Mathew (my batchmate) in 1962 were the brave souls before me after George Cherian in 1957. In 1963, two candidates who were not selected for the MS degree programme were offered the opportunity to join for the MD General

Medicine and they accepted. So for the first time in many years, there were three candidates for MD General Medicine.

Accommodation for junior doctors in the Hospital Campus was a problem. The Lady Internes Quarters, a priority of Dr. Hilda Lazarus, was completed in 1954, but accommodation for men doctors was very limited on the Hospital Campus. The Small Bungalow where the Occupational Therapy and Haematology block now stands and the dilapidated Red House (where the Hospital Canteen is now) had rooms where men doctors stayed. The completion of the first floor of the new OPD block in 1959 provided a block of rooms over the Casualty (now occupied by the Dental Department) for the men doctors. One of Dr. Carman's priorities was good accommodation for the men doctors and in January 1962 the Men Internes Quarters was completed with what then was considered luxurious single rooms with attached toilets. Very soon, all the groundfloor rooms were occupied by young married couples. This accommodation was a great boon as I can vouch after having moved in to room 116 on the groundfloor of MIQ after marriage in April 1962.

The 1960s was a good time to be young and a postgraduate student at CMCV. The faculty was being built up by recruiting young Indians with postgraduate qualifications mostly obtained in India. Vellore provided an excellent opportunity to establish yourselves if you had postgraduate qualifications and wanted to work and grow with a Christian academic institution.

Aunt Ida passes away

Aunt Ida would have completed ninety years on December 9, 1960. She had been frail for at least 5 years and in a wheelchair for two years, spending the warmer months in Kodaikanal at her lovely home Hill Top, coming down to Vellore in the cooler months including Christmas and the New Year. On 26 of May, 1960 she passed away peacefully at Kodaikanal. A pall of gloom enveloped Vellore when the news was flashed. Her body was brought overnight to Vellore and the town virtually shut down for a day when after a service on the hospital lawn the body was taken in procession to the cemetery through the town. Many joined the funeral procession so that when the body reached the cemetery, the end of the procession had not left the Hospital lawn 4 km away. She was considered a saint or mother by many in the town and the outpour of grief was genuine. Fortunately, the institution that she had founded had strong roots and sixty years later is still alive and vibrant as she would have wished, continuing to heal patients and train young women and men in the spirit of Christ.

Many of us staff, students and others who followed her body in the long walk from the hospital to the cemetery vowed that the inspiration that she had given and traditions established over the many years she was with us should be preserved and built upon as a living memorial to her inspiring life. It was fortunate that by 1960 a strong Indian faculty and staff had been built up, not by chance but by a deliberate effort to indigenise the Institution. It was equally important that the faculty and staff were conscious that maintaining tradition entailed active participation in the life of this Christian Institution. Maintaining the Christian character of the College involved conscious effort to keep the centrality of Christ in the life of the community. This was brought to focus about three years after her death when one of our faculty had serious postpartum problems and saving her life involved the entire community with continuous prayer in the Hospital chapel for over two weeks, during which time the staff donated over 70 bottles of blood for her. That was a team effort that has characterised CMCV in times of trouble and stress. However, we continue to feel the void.

The Jubilee was celebrated in 1960, and the Institution was able to purchase a large plot of ground contiguous to the Hospital Campus to the east where residences for staff and students were built. Residential accommodation on the Hospital Campus was always limited and the many residences built during the 60s were replaced by high rise buildings thirty years later still not satisfying the demand for on–campus accommodation. This will always continue to be a challenge as the Institution grows in response to felt needs.

The Carman Era concludes

1960 to 1967 was a period of growth and stabilisation. The clinical and pre–clinical undergraduate teaching departments were well established and had adequate staff with a heavy teaching load. Anatomy, Physiology, Biochemistry, Pharmacology and Community Medicine were in the College Campus. Apart from the Women's and Men's Hostels on the College Campus many faculty houses came up. The Department of Psychiatry and the Rehabilitation Institute were established on extensions of the campus. The Community Medicine Department and the Rural Hospital were also on the campus. The new out–patient block with the Norman Auditorium and the Norman Institute of Pathology on the top floor, were built with generous grants from the Norman Foundation in Australia. The top floor of the out–patient block housed the department of Pathology while Microbiology was on the top two floors of the old out–patient block with Blood Bank on the ground floor and administrative offices in between.

It was a time of consolidation in the College with many young postgraduates recruited to the faculty. All such recruits were encouraged to take study leave up to three years for enhancing their knowledge and skills. When Dr. John Carman retired from the Institution after thirteen years of service, he had placed the Institution in a position of strength. Mrs. Carman served as the Treasurer during most of these years and her faithful stewardship was a major factor in the growth and strengthening of the Institution. One of her major contributions was identifying and training Mr. CC Jacob to take over as the Treasurer from her. Mr. Jacob served CMCV faithfully till 1990 and was a major factor in the growth and stability of the Institution where finances were always limited.

Dr. Carman built a strong and cohesive administrative team to carry on after his retirement. Dr. Jacob Chandy, Principal, Dr. Daniel Isaac, Medical Superintendent, Miss Aleyamma Kuruvilla, Dean College of Nursing, Miss Anna Jacob Nursing Superintendent and Rev. A S S Avarirayan, General Superintendent were this team. Dr. JKG Webb was Deputy Director and was selected as Director to succeed Dr. Carman.

Chapter 8

Storm Clouds Gather 1967 to 1974

JKG Webb, KG Koshy and LBM Joseph

The transition from the Carman era to that of John Webb was smooth as he was familiar with ongoing work as Deputy Director. Dr. KG Koshy was appointed as Deputy Director with no change in any of the other Administrative Officers. The Institution had grown from a small missionary establishment to one of the largest teaching Hospitals and Medical Colleges in India. Unlike the early days of Aunt Ida working with just the help of Naomi, there was a large number of non-medical staff, as well as Medical and Nursing professionals. The Medical and Nursing staff were more in number, compared to other Medical colleges of similar student intake for two reasons. Firstly the finances for the College was maintained by the income from the excellent clinical services in the Hospital. The Institution had therefore recruited the optimum staff necessary for clinical services and not just the minimum staff necessary for University recognition as a college. Secondly being situated in a small town far away from major urban centers all expertise for running the College and Hospital, medical and non-medical, effectively had to be available in house.

The faculty predominantly Christian, was a mixture of Missionaries from UK and USA and Australia supplemented by recruits mainly from graduates and postgraduates of the Institution. The number of Overseas Missionaries on the staff gradually decreased and their positions taken up by well qualified Indians. The Nurses, except for a few Missionaries, were almost all Graduates and Post-graduates of Vellore. Locally recruited staff, many from the local Christian community, provided the support services for the Institution. The support staff were reasonably educated, since from the inception the Institution insisted on defined minimum educational standards for each level of appointment. The Faculty at Vellore had accepted that their emoluments would not be comparable to that even of their Indian peers in State Government Medical Colleges. These Government Colleges also permitted private practice which provided the bulk of the Faculty income. The non-monetary rewards of being Faculty at CMC Vellore were not quantifiable but very satisfying for most of the Faculty. While Faculty salaries were 50% or less of what it was at the All India Institute of Medical Sciences (AIIMS) New Delhi, the Institution tried to pay salaries comparable to that of the State Government Medical Services to the other staff. However there were constant demands from these staff for salary increases.

In the middle of the last century given these circumstances the growth of a Labour Union in the Institution was inevitable. Local Political Parties, who had been kept strictly at arms length by the Administration, saw this as an opportunity to have a say in the affairs of the Institution by stirring the pot. The party ruling the state became the Godfather of the Union which had the largest number of members, the CMC Vellore Employees Union, registered as NAT 29 with the Labour Department.

Some of the faculty, both from India and abroad, welcomed this development and felt the growth of a responsible Labour Union would be good for the Institution. In fact a few of them even attended the inaugural meeting of the Union. In their socialistic idealism they forgot that Labour Unions are usually concerned only about the welfare and wealth of their leaders and related Politicians! The majority of the Faculty were however worried that a Labour union controlled by local politicians would lead to indiscipline and unrest, most undesirable in a patient care Institution.

Two extracts from Council minutes illustrate the situation.

"The General Superintendent has referred briefly in his report to the fact that a Union of Class III and IV workers has been formed and registered and that in the past two months 2 lightning strikes have taken place. It is clear that the formation of a Union is to be expected today in an institution of our size. This Union has to be recognized and I have during this past week taken steps to set up a committee which will include representatives elected from the staff eligible for Union membership as well as members nominated by me. This committee will consider all matters raised by the Union, and will thus constitute a channel of communication between the staff and the administration. I am hopeful that through this committee acceptable ways of handling· future problems will be found. It is obvious that we face difficulties, but no more than at all stages of our history. Our strength lies in the quality of our staff which would be hard to match in any other institution. But more than this, our strength rests in the hands of God, a strength available to us in so far as we consciously trust Him. And ultimately it is the fact that we do have this sense that He has guided in the past, and that He guides us now,

over-ruling our mistakes and correcting our misunderstandings, that provides the surest ground for confidence in the future of this great institution." (Council Minutes, September 1968, Page 90, last para of Directors report)

The pressure from the Union was felt by the Staff and even by the Council as reflected in this report by the Council Chair to the same Council meeting.

"Arising out of the concluding.paragraph of the Director's Report, having reference to the formation and registration of a Union of workers of the Institution, the Chairman of the meeting reported to the Council that he had received on the evening of 11-9-68 in the Director's Office, when the Director and the Dy. Director (Dr K. G. Koshy) were also present, a deputation of Staff constituting ten of the office bearers of the Union. They presented him a printed Memorandum containing matters they desired to represent to the Administration and which they wanted conveyed to the meeting of the Council. The Acting-Chairman explained that he had agreed to read out the Memorandum to the Council, and accordingly read it out. He mentioned that his meeting with the Union representatives took place in a cordial atmosphere and had concluded with prayer and the benediction. The Director on his side, and the Union representatives on their side, appreciated that mere technicalities (pending recognition of the Union), would not impede communication with the Union. The Union representatives also agreed not to press some of their demands, while the Director referred to the steps he had taken (as mentioned in the last paragraph of his annual Report to the Council which forms Appendix A hereto) to set up a Committee which will include representatives elected from the staff eligible for Union membership as well as members nominated by him'

(Director) and 'which will consider all matters raised by the Union and will thus constitute a channel of communication between the staff and the administration. "

The Union was registered by the local labour Officer, but the Institution did not formally recognise it or provide privileges a Union enjoys in an industrial establishment. The Institutions relationship with the Union started on a note of cordiality and mutual respect hoping to work together for the good of both the parties. Unfortunately it rapidly became an adversarial relationship as it became clear to the Faculty and Administration that the motives driving the Union leadership was not the welfare of the employees and the Institution but self-aggrandisement of individual leaders. In 1974 the involvement of the elder brother of the Union leader, the only member of the faculty from the town of Vellore, in a case of corruption regarding admission to the MBBS program resulted in a major confrontation leading to a 70 day strike by the union, of which more later.

In 1973 Dr. KG Koshy, the Director reported to the Council:

'There were very many problems in our relationship with our employees. I had reported to you last year about the strike we had in July 1972. Except for a few problems that arose during the post-strike period, discussion with the Union representatives were free and cordial. They had free access to the Personnel Manager and the Assistant Personnel Officer and most of the problems were settled by them. Problems which could not be dealt with by them were discussed at the meetings of the Negotiating Committee. There were stoppages of work by various sections of employees for short periods, but these were settled without delay. In May 1973 as certain decisions made by the administration were not acceptable to some sections of

the employees there were tense situations. By tactful handling and with the help of the Mediation Body these disputes were settled and normalcy restored. The Personnel Department has been a great source of help in dealing with the various problems which have arisen during the year. We have to realise that good staff relationship is absolutely necessary for the institution to be viable and fulfil its role in service, training and research. I do hope that in the years to come all employees in the institution will realise the purpose of the institution and the importance of all sections respecting each other's right and working together to witness for the Master". Council Min Oct 1973. Director's Report Pages78,79.

John Webb as Director when the Union started adopted a policy of pandering to the Union's demands where procrastination did not help. When he suddenly resigned and returned to UK in the latter half of 1971 KG Koshy inherited the legacy of Union relationship started by him. Shanthi Fenn took over the Principals office from KG Koshy and scrupulously confined himself to student affairs and relationship with the University. Although he was the second in seniority in the Administration and the head of a Surgical Unit he tried to keep away as far as possible from all Union related problems.

Life in the College

A generational Change occurred in `1967 when two senior members of the faculty Dr. KI Vythilingam, Professor of Medicine and Cardiology and Prof Ida B Scudder, Professor of Radiology, as well as Dr and Mrs Carman who had contributed to the growth and development of the Institution formally retired. KIV belonged to the second batch of diploma Medical students and through her long service at Vellore was sponsored by the Institution to obtain MBBS and MD Degrees from the Madras University. She was the first Alumna to become Professor of Medicine at Vellore and then start a new specialty, the Department, Cardiology. She rose to be the doyen of Cardiology in India. I remember assisting her in a cardiac catheterisation in the X-ray Department as a Medical postgraduate student and being impressed by her skilful dexterity in this then pioneering venture. She was joined by two of the Alumni, George Cherian, the first to obtain DM in Cardiology from Vellore and IP Sukumar, trained abroad in Paediatric Cardiology. Though the Institution missed this distinguished daughter when she superannuated, she had trained her colleagues so well that professionally her absence did not make a dent in the services. George and IPS took the department to greater heights.

Prof Ida B Scudder, Aunt Ida's niece, was the second and last of the Scudders to serve Vellore. As a child she was thrilled and inspired by the life of dedicated service of her Aunt, became a doctor and came to work with her in 1931. Although what she wanted to do was to work with sick children, she served the Institution wherever she was asked to. When immediately on arrival in India she was undergoing language school in Kodaikanal, she was urgently called to Vellore to take charge of the ENT Department, a specialty she had no experience of! Before she finally found her specialty of Radiology, responding to urgent needs of the hospital, she had worked in Paediatrics, Eye, Ear Nose and Throat, Medicine and Gynaecology and Obstetrics! In 1934 when Aunt Ida returning from furlough brought Radium needles and the first X-ray therapy machine, IdaB was asked to take charge. It was decided that in preparation for starting the MBBS program, as part of acquiring qualified

Faculty, she would pass the Radiology examinations in UK, as US qualifications were not then recognised by the University. It is a measure of her dedication to Vellore that she spent 3 years in UK, passed the examinations and came back just as the Second World War started.   As the last Scudder at Vellore IdaB was an inspirational focal point for the students and the staff and was always available to serve as acting administrator in any post where the incumbent was temporarily absent. An example of her ability and firmness was shown when she called a brilliant young clinician who insisted on doing late night rounds with the lady House staff to her office. When she suggested to the Clinician that this was not quite appropriate, he was outraged that she dared to advise him and threatened to resign if she did not apologise. Quietly IdaB offered him a sheet of paper, requested his letter of resignation and accepted it on the spot!

IdaB excelled not only in her chosen specialty, Radiology, and the many roles she played as an Administrator, but also in continuing the tradition of the Roadside clinic started by Aunt Ida. For many years she was in charge of the Friday Odugathoor Roadside. Students looked forward to the opportunity to go with her and her team for a day. The roadside experience gave the students an opportunity to learn how to deal with the many clinical problems in rural areas with minimal facilities. They also learnt from the many patients with leprosy and its myriad manifestations not easily found in the Hospital. After the last stop at the Odugathoor market they would return to the Hostel late in the evening knowing they had helped the sick and the suffering where facilities were not available.   Although at its peak there were five roadside clinics, one each day of the week, by mid-1950 it had come down to two, the Chittoor Roadside on Wednesdays with MD Graham and Odugathoor on Fridays with IdaB. When Roadside clinics were started, it was a much needed pioneering endeavour helping the rural poor with limited access to health care and was considered a flagship program of CMCV. But the situation was changing and by the late sixties a Government Primary Health Center was opened in Odugathoor and a policy decision was made to close the Roadside activity. It is significant that the recent expansion of clinical and diagnostic facilities into the Chittoor District of Andhra Pradesh is located almost on the spot where the Gudipala Hut stop, the second one on the Chittoor Roadside used to be. Fifty years in the future!

The Institution celebrated the Centenary of the birth of Aunt Ida in 1970. Four years prior to this work on the Scudder Auditorium, a memorial to Aunt Ida, was completed. The beautiful building was planned by Architect Mr. Bennet Pithavadian and most of the funds for the building were raised by the Scudder family who were well represented at the inauguration in 1966. This 1000 seat Auditorium, the outdoor stage and spacious Hall, are a great asset and has significantly enhanced the social and cultural life on the campus. It has also been the venue of several all India Conferences of specialist Medical Societies proving its value in Medical education. Dr Ida B Scudder came back from retirement for the inauguration.

The low salaries of the staff were a concern all through this period. The social concern of the Institution was shown by the salaries of the lower paid staff being revised upwards, albeit by small amounts, at each council meeting while the Faculty salaries were revised only at longer intervals. The worry was that all expenditure, including salaries, were from money earned by patient care. The Faculty and administration were wary of increasing the charge to the patient at frequent (six monthly) intervals and worried whether we would choke off patient flow with increased rates. In the 1960's CMCV saw itself as a hospital for middle class patients with a few rich patients coming for specialised care. The earnings from the paying patients met the cost of the considerable amount of charity work for the poor. The policy decision that the Institution should earn its keep by providing high quality services to outpatients as well as to those admitted, and use the money earned thereby to pay salaries and run the Institution was never formally discussed and adopted. By the mid 1960's a consensus regarding this strategy had come about and it was accepted that the number of private ward beds should approximately be one third of the total beds. Gradually it became clear that it was not just the scientific quality of our services that attracted patients to Vellore but that the totality of the experience, the empathy of all staff and the patient centeredness of the Institution were the key to our success as a hospital. It was remarkable how this tradition based on Christ centeredness grew and became the ethos of Vellore.

Central to this was the conscious effort of each faculty to try and envisage what Dr. Scudder would have done in any situation, never forgetting that she started clinical service before education and that while she started a Compounder training program three years later it was another six years before nursing education was formalised and almost ten more years before Medical student training started. The centrality of the quality and compassion expressed through our services in the Hospital to the development and growth of the Institution and the quality of Medical education, was soon recognised by all the staff, not just the medical and nursing. Unfortunately a few local members on the staff were not prepared to give primacy to the patients and the Institution and tried to establish themselves as powers to be feared, by fomenting trouble through the Union.

Administrative timidity encourages Union Indiscipline

What stands out to those of us who were on the staff between the latter half of the sixties and mid-seventies is the tremendous tolerance and forbearance shown by the Administration of the arrogant behaviour of the Union leaders. The Faculty and Administration were hopeful at the start of the Union that it was likely to ensure smooth functioning of the Institution with cordial relationship between the Administration, Faculty and the staff represented by the Union. Two things became clear very soon. Majority of the staff were not interested in becoming members of the Union. They were quite content with their relationship with their peers in their own Departments and confident that the Departmental Faculty and the Head would look after their best interests. They were not prepared to trust the so called Union leaders and leave their future welfare in their hands. This upset the Union as they expected all staff to pay Union dues but only less than 30% actually did so. The Union requested the Administration to collect the dues compulsorily from all non-medical and non-nursing staff. Of course there was no way the Administration was going to do this and there was no way the Union could compel them to their will. The majority of the staff was happy that their salaries were received in full and that union dues were not deducted compulsorily!

The Union actually was started by a few of the local members of the staff in the clerical grade to assume and assert leadership and gain a sense of power. Less than a handful of the Faculty who felt frustrated that they were not selected for administrative responsibilities supported and instigated them behind the scene. The vast majority of the Faculty and more than 80% of the staff were only interested that they should be able to continue to teach the students and offer the best of services to the patients in a calm and serene atmosphere. Unfortunately the leaders of the Union saw that the only way they could make an impact and gain prominence was by creating trouble in the Institution. To do this they recruited all the trouble makers in the institution as members and also allied with outside political elements. John Webb was the Director, Daniel Isaac the Medical Superintendent and Jacob Chandy the Principal in 1968 when the Union was first registered. While the Director and the Medical Superintendent were willing for dialogue with the Union, the Principal and the majority of the Faculty were keen that maintenance of strict discipline in the Institution was essential for optimum patient care.

The Director, John Webb, offered free access to him for the leaders of the Union and it became the accepted norm that the Union leaders and their trouble making colleagues could barge in to the Director's office with their demands, reasonable or otherwise (mostly the latter) whenever they felt like it. The Principal was the only one who resisted this and he became the focal point of their hatred and they started on a campaign of vilification, which unfortunately took on a linguistic colour. Jacob Chandy left for a Sabbatical year with the Christian Medical Commission of the World Council of Churches in Geneva in 1970. During this time the University reiterated that the normal age of retirement was 60, although faculty could continue till the age of 65 with yearly permission from the University. This actually was not a new rule but only a reiteration of the existing provisions. Webb however interpreted this reiteration as a new rule and informed Jacob Chandy that his appointment was terminated and got his house on the campus vacated at short notice. Mrs Chandy had to pack and leave as the Director was insistent on getting the house back! As Jacob Chandy says in his autobiography, he was fully aware of the rules of the University and knew that Webb's interpretation was wrong. However as a disciplined member of the staff he did not contest the Director's wrong decision. While the Institution lost the services of a nationally and Internationally reputed pioneer in Neurosurgery and an excellent Administrator, Jacob Chandy was not personally harmed as he had a very successful career in practice in Kerala with financial rewards unimaginable while serving in Vellore! He also made a significant contribution to the Medical Board of the Church of South India Madhya Kerala Diocese as its Chair and significantly improved the service of their Hospitals. This unceremonious "sacking" of Jacob Chandy was the worst example of a lack of administrative judgement by John Webb.

Soon after this John Webb was offered a Professorship in Paediatrics in London and accepting this he resigned from Vellore. KG Koshy, Professor of Community Medicine, a much loved teacher who was the then Principal was selected to be the next Director from the latter half of 1971 and Dr Shanthi Fenn, Professor of Surgery and Head Surgery Unit II, was appointed as Principal. At the same time Dr. LBM Joseph Professor of Surgery and Head of Surgery Unit III was asked to be Acting Medical Superintendent as Dr Daniel Isaac, the full time Medical Superintendent was on Sabbatical leave working as the Secretary of the Christian Medical Association of India. These changes in the Senior Administration coincided with increased Union activity. The Union soon discovered that if Webb had been willing to succumb to their demands KG was equally submissive and non-assertive. The only one who resisted the Union's adventurism and tried to insist on discipline being maintained in the hospital was LBM.

I was away on a year and a half of study leave from April 1970 to September 1971, and on return just before John Webb's resignation, found a rather disturbed Institution where a number of the support staff were no longer interested in their work and pursued an agitational approach to impose their will on the Administration. While individual Faculty maintained their patient care standards, the overall quality of patient care had deteriorated. The Administration was passively reactive to events and not proactive in guiding the faculty, staff and students into an envisioned future. It was obvious that the Director did not have a clear vision of the future and that the future was bleak unless the Faculty clearly articulated a vision and stood with a person who was willing to lead to that future. The majority of the faculty soon realised that the only possible leader capable of doing this was Dr. LBM Joseph.

The Koshy years were marked by turbulent indiscipline in the Hospital and rumours of corruption gradually becoming a way of life for many in the Institution. The problems at Vellore due to the indiscipline and power hunger of the Union leaders continued. Indiscipline, threats of, and actual strikes and petty corruption by the lower paid employees became the norm. The administration was unable to control the indiscipline of the Union. The quality of patient care began to suffer due to this.

It is difficult for those who did not live through this at Vellore to feel the atmosphere in the Institution during this period.

It is not an exaggeration to say that the vast majority of the Faculty were working in Vellore because of their commitment as Christians to the healing Ministry of Christ. Almost 90% of the Faculty were and are Christian and it is true to say that all of them could command a job in any Institution in India at several times the salary they earned at Vellore. Almost all the Faculty have worked abroad during periods of study leave and most of them have been offered positions in the Departments where they trained. My wife and I spent a year and a half in 1970-71 at Boston University School of Medicine on study leave. When we were getting ready to come back to Vellore we were given tempting offers to stay on. Two years later I was invited to go back and head the Department of Gastroenterology where I trained. Very few have accepted such offers, but all have managed to keep good relationships with those institutions and have later on obtained training opportunities for their students and colleagues! By and large it would be correct to say that the Faculty are serving at Vellore because they have been called to do so. For the majority of Faculty it is a commitment to serve in the healing ministry of Christ rather than a career in the premier Medical College in the Country. Many in the faculty began to examine what their response should be if the discipline in the Institution did not improve. They were looking for a leader who could guide them out of the mess.

Towards a new paradigm of Administration.

KG Koshy's term as Director was ending in March 1974. The Council appointed a Nomination Committee to choose the next Director at the end of 1972 so that the person selected could have administrative training at the Indian Institute of Management, Ahmedabad. The consultations, the Committee had with the faculty clearly indicated that what was needed was a person who would re-establish discipline in the Institution. After extensive consultations the committee chose Prof. LBM Joseph, Professor of Surgery and Head Surgery Unit 3 for this position against the bitter and at times violent opposition of the Labour Union. The vast majority of the Faculty welcomed this choice and were sure he would offer the necessary leadership and develop a new paradigm of administration. LBM went for a tailored program in administration at the Indian Institute of Management (IIM) at Ahmedabad. One or two of the Senior Faculty felt that in choosing LBM their claims were overlooked and they became quite unhappy.

In May 1974 soon after LBM returned from IIM Ahmedabad and took over as Director from KG Koshy, information was received by the Institution alleging serious corruption in the MBBS selection for that year. This was through a pseudonymous letter received by the Chaplain requesting information on how next year the letter writer could ensure the admission of his daughter to the MBBS course as was done in the case of Miss X, her room-mate in their College Hostel, who had been called for interview in 1974 June? Details of who should be contacted and to whom the money should be paid were requested! Immediate confidential investigation by the Director and Principal found evidence that two candidates, both from outside India had been given marks much more than their actual entrance examination answer papers deserved. Based on these false marks they both had been called for interview from among the open candidates. The call for interview of these two candidates were cancelled and a detailed investigation was started. During the investigation two of the clerical staff in the Registrar's Office involved in the selection confessed and implicated two other clerical staff and a Faculty member Dr Alpheus Joseph, Reader in ENT. Unfortunately Alpheus happened to be the elder brother of the leader of the employees union and also the only person from Vellore on the Faculty. Based on the evidence gathered by the internal enquiry a detailed external enquiry was conducted by a retired District and Sessions Judge of impeccable reputation who found Alpheus and four clerical staff guilty as charged.

From the time the guilty were identified the Union came into the picture demanding that no action should be taken on any of them, especially Alpheus. The union was supported in this demand by only three out of over a hundred senior Faculty. The Institution was in turmoil with polarisation of the Faculty, the three senior staff along with the Union demanding that no further action was taken. The majority of the Faculty were in favour of discipline and clear that this kind of corruption demanded the ultimate punishment, dismissal from the Institution.   The three dissident Faculty and the Union recruited the help of local politicians of the Party in power in the state and influenced the Collector, the highest District Official, and the senior members of the political party in power in the State to get them on their side.

At the same time there were eighteen other employees under suspension pending enquiry on charges of violence and destruction of property. These charges were serious and would invite the punishment up to dismissal if proven. The Union was adamant that no enquiry should be held. Since Alpheus was a Council appointee the entire disciplinary issues were placed before the Council at its meeting in October 1974. The Union attempted to intimidate the Council also without success. After careful examination of all the facts the Council concurred with the decision to terminate the employment of the five individuals who were proven to have been involved in the corruption about MBBS admission and to hold appropriate enquiries on the others who were not Council Appointees. The Council left it to the judgement of the Director to decide when action should be taken, in consultation with Dr. MA Thangaraj, the Chair of the Council, a senior Educationists and Principal of the American College Madurai. The MBBS selection corruption problems are mentioned in the directors report to the October 1974 Council. However it is interesting that the Principal in reporting on the MBBS Selection 1974 to the Council does not mention this issue at all!

The atmosphere in the College and Hospital was tense and there was a sense of impending problems in the air. The administration was worried that the Union had indulged in violence against members of staff who did not agree with their tactics of violence and intimidation. The guilt of Dr.Alpheus Joseph and his assistants had been proven beyond doubt by the independent enquiry. There were also at least another 18 members of the Union against whom serious misconduct had been proven. The findings against them merited dismissal as punishment.

In December 1974 it was decided to hold an enquiry regarding the 18 staff under suspension for serious indiscipline and notice was given that the enquiry was to begin on Monday, January 6, 1975. At 9PM on Sunday January 5 1975 the Union went on strike and it was clear that this was to prevent the enquiry proposed for the next day. There was intimidation of and violence against the staff working that night and against the Security Officer, Mr Balraj Epiphany. The Administrative Officers managed to reach the Hospital past midnight and tried to bring about a semblance of order with the help of the Police and the District Administration. What started on the January 5 went on for the next seventy days and nearly brought Christian Medical College Vellore to a standstill.

Chapter 9

The Seventy Day Strike January 5 – March 15, 1975

Dr. LBM Joseph

The Institution was unfortunately accustomed to a turbulent labour relationship, occasional gheraos, strikes for a day or two and a generally uncertain atmosphere by the end of 1974. Dismissal of Alpheus Joseph and his four fellow conspirators involved in the admissions corruption in 1974 was confirmed by the Council in October 1974, leaving the timing of the action to the Director, LBM Joseph in consultation with the Council Chair. There were also another 15 individuals in the clerical and attender grade charged with major indiscipline awaiting detailed enquiry by an enquiry committee appointed by the Council. The implementation of any external enquiry and other disciplinary action was held in abeyance knowing that it would lead to strikes and other problems, as all involved members of the militant trade union.

Dr. MA Thangaraj the then Principal of the American College, Madurai was the Council Chair. He was an experienced educationist and administrator and deeply committed to the Institution and always available for advice and consultation. On his advice it was decided to start the enquiry by a retired District Judge on Monday January 6, 1975 and notice was given to the employees concerned to be present for the enquiry at 9.00AM. The Union wrote to the Director that they had advised the concerned staff not to attend the enquiry. They actually went on strike at around 9.00PM on the night of Sunday January 5 to try and ensure that there would be no enquiry on the sixth.

Sunday is a relatively quiet day in the Hospital and most of the Faculty and Administrators after a brief morning round would be at home, most of them staying at the College campus. As soon as the information on the strike was received, the Director requested the Collector and the Superintendent of Police to provide Police protection for the patients and those looking after them in the Hospital. The Director and several senior Faculty managed to reach the Hospital by about midnight and found the Hospital in darkness with no staff in the Blood Bank or Pharmacy as they had been chased out by the striking workers. The ward staff were harassed by the striking workers who wanted the Nursing Sisters and House Staff to leave their place of duty. Gangs of strikers were roaming the Hospital campus threatening all who worked and also patient relatives. In fact an elderly Gentleman wheeling an oxygen cylinder for his sick son was assaulted by the striking workers. The Police were by and large passive bystanders during this time. By early morning skeletal staff to keep the Blood Bank and Pharmacy working were available. House staff stayed in all wards to look after patients as it was difficult to find attenders to call Doctors on duty.

Monday January 6th and Tuesday the 7th were rather chaotic days with Nurses and Doctors taking care of the admitted patients and discharging as many of them as possible. Emergency patients were seen and laboratories were functional. By Tuesday evening the Police agreed to keep striking workers out of the Hospital campus and the Nursing and House staff were able to look after their patients better. Ways were found for those who wanted to work to come to the campus through some of the Houses in Thottapalayam at the back of the campus. Faculty and other senior staff came through the main gate with the strikers jeering them especially the ladies. This prompted one of the Senior Lady staff to quip that it was good they didn't understand what was shouted at them in Tamil as they walked by, although they knew it was not complimentary!

It was clear that the strike had been called to prevent an enquiry on the charge sheeted staff. Since there were several other enquiries scheduled to be held, it was likely that a cycle of strikes to prevent enquiries would be standard operating procedure for the Labour Union. The Union started this strike without notice and had also not made any demands or raised disputes with the Administration. It was an illegal strike as defined in labour laws. The Director Dr. LBM Joseph, in consultation with the Council Chair therefore decided that since preliminary in-house enquiry had established the clear guilt of these individuals it would be best to dismiss them from service. The informal understanding that the proposed dismissal of the five found guilty of the admission malpractices would be held in abeyance was also no longer binding as the Union had already started a strike without apparent provocation. Therefore on Wednesday January 8, 1975 the five employees including Dr Alpheus Joseph and the 15 against whom the enquiry was proposed were dismissed from service. Orders of dismissal were sent to their residential addresses by Registered post acknowledgement due as well as by certificate of posting and copies posted on the notice boards in their respective departments as well as the notice boards of the appointing authorities. The registered letters came back as not deliverable, but the letters under certificate of posting were not returned and presumed to be delivered.

The Administration also refused to have any further discussions with the striking employees and requested the Collector to ensure protection for patients and all who wanted to work. It became clear that only a proportion of the Attenders and Clerical staff were supporting the strike. The hardcore Union members were less than hundred, but by coercive methods they managed to have about a thousand of the lower paid employees join them. Since from the third day of the strike the Police ensured that striking employees were kept out of the campus it was possible to continue the work of the Hospital. The few who came to the outpatients were seen, any who needed admission were admitted and some non-emergency surgical procedures were done. The Hospital was working at about a fifth of its capacity, although it was less than a thousand of the four thousand or so employees who were on strike.

The organiser and Secretary of the Union was Jayakaran Joseph, a clerical staff in a project in the ENT Department. He was the younger brother of Dr Alpheus Joseph, the only Faculty from the town in the Institution, who had been found guilty in the admission corruption. Jayakaran was on study leave in the USA with financial support from the Institution when the strike started. He came back to Vellore by the end of the first week of the strike, without permission from the Institution with the excuse of a death in the family! The demand of the striking workers by that time was that Dr Alpheus Joseph and the five guilty of corruption in that years admission to the MBBS program, as well as the 15 other employees terminated on January 8th should be reinstated unconditionally. This of course was an issue that came up after the strike was started by them to prevent an enquiry into the issue.

The Administration and the loyal staff were not prepared to even discuss this issue with the Union or the striking workers. Jayakaran found that he was not able to achieve anything to further the cause of his brother and returned to USA after a week in Vellore. The strike dragged on with no end in sight. The Collector and the Police had the situation under control and it was possible for the vast majority of the Faculty as well as the Medical and Nursing staff to come to work. Around forty per cent of the clerical and attender staff also were reporting for work and the Hospital services functioned reasonably well although patients coming for care were few. The majority of the Administration and the Faculty were determined to continue to work as well as they could and all who came to the Institution for care were looked after although the inpatient strength was much reduced.

Professor and Head of Radiodiagnosis, Professor and Head of the Anaesthesiology and Professor and Head of Radiation Therapy were the only three among over a hundred Senior faculty who were openly sympathetic to Alpheus and the Union who was supporting him. Each one of them in succession sat for 12 hours of hunger strike at a tent put up just outside the entrance gate of the Hospital on 23rd, 24th and 25th of January.

While they sat on hunger strike they made no demands and we still do not know what their demands were! It was presumed that it was in sympathy with the striking workers who made much of them and sat with them in the tent but they were ignored by the rest of the Senior Faculty, the Administration and the loyal workers. Their twelve hour fasting had no apparent impact on the situation.

The frustration of the striking workers at this drawn out strike was palpable and every day a few workers left the strikers and reported for duty. This frustration increased when the salary for January was paid to all working staff on January 25th, a few days in advance of the usual date of payment on the last day of the month. It was made clear that the policy was 'No work, no pay' knowing that the majority of workers had no reserve and were dependent on their salaries for day to day expenses. The timely payment of salary to all working employees was a major blow to striking employees. The Union of course had no resources to pay anything to those on strike! A further action that caused consternation to the leaders of the strike was two of the 15 other employees who were terminated on January 8th being reinstated after a review by the Executive Committee who determined that their misdemeanours were of lesser gravity. This clearly showed to all staff that the charges of vindictiveness against the Institution was not really sustainable.

The three dissident Senior faculty used all their influence to persuade the political party in power in the state, to put pressure on the Administration to reinstate the dismissed staff and the five guilty of admission corruption and thereby bring the strike to an end. The Administration, the vast majority of the senior Faculty and the loyal staff were clear that any lenience on the part of the Institution would make maintenance of discipline impossible and no concessions could be made. This position was made clear to the Government through the Vellore Collector.

The State Government increased the pressure on the Institution in a variety of ways. Several loyal workers were arrested including the acting head of Pharmacy Services. Late one night an unruly crowd including striking workers and others came to the College campus and tried to attack the house of one of the Senior Faculty, but when he came out to confront them they ran away, suggesting they had little stomach for what their leaders was putting them up to! The water supply to the Hospital campus was temporarily disrupted by cutting the pipe. There were also threats that the compound wall along the main highway at the front of the Hospital was encroaching and would be pulled down. In fact the Institution was able to show that the Highway was actually encroaching on the Hospital property and several decades earlier this encroachment had been regularised.

Local leaders tried to mediate on behalf of the striking workers and the letter dated March 8, 1975 quoted below addressed to some of them by the Director clearly outlines the position of the Institution.

March 8, 1975

To:

Sri MP Sarathi

Sri Lalalajapathi

Sri Jeevarathna Mudaliar /

and all other friends of the Christian Medical College and Hospital, Vellore

Dear Sirs/Friends:

At the outset my colleagues and I would like to express our heartfelt gratitude to all of you for giving us so much of your valuable time for prolonged discussions on more than one occasion, and on Wednesday, 5th March. 1975 in the Director's Office of the Christian Medical College and Hospital.

More so, your presence and efforts were an expression of your deep love for the Christian Medical College and Hospital and its staff, and a genuine and sincere anxiety that the welfare of the hospital should be maintained at all costs, and that no harm should come to the institution, however difficult the present situation may be.

Many of us could sense this genuine affection and concern and we are very grateful. Your association with this institution is perhaps much longer than many of us who have come only about 20 and odd years ago. You have seen the growth of this institution, as citizens of this town, for several decades and you have received inspiration from its Founder, Doctor Ida Scudder. You have also taken pride that this nationally and internationally famous institution is situated in this historical town of Vellore and that by its service has attracted hundreds and thousands of patients from within our beloved country and also from other neighbouring countries.

My colleagues and I, in our travels throughout the world, have met many people for whom Vellore is India. They have heard of the name of no other town in India, except Vellore and this must justifiably give you pride as the leading citizens of this town of

Vellore. In addition to seeing the growth of this institution, of understanding the richness of its service of taking pride in its achievements, you have also taken a share in its difficulties and you are anxious to help in this situation. Again, my colleagues and I, express our grateful thanks to you.

I need not go into the history of the present difficulties. You are all well familiar with them. Moreover, you are familiar with the history of events which have taken place in this institution over the last six or seven years. The society throughout the world is changing and in this changing concept the attitudes of some members of staff have also changed, leading on to agitational type of activities. It is unfortunate that these types of agitational activities should be in a social organisation like a hospital where there are hundreds of patients, whose welfare is the prime concern of every staff member. Also these agitational activities have been at the expense of patients who have been held as ransom in situations like the present strike. Fortunately, devotion and dedication to Patients of large numbers of doctors and nurses, technicians and other loyal workers has prevented patient care being used as a ransom for achieving ends through agitation. ·

Again, I repeat, Sirs, it is not necessary to dwell on the details of the present situation. However, it may be that you do not know that in addition to the strikes and other methods of agitational activities, there have been many, many unpublicised incidents of indiscipline which have eroded into the very fibre and moral structure of this organisation. To give you examples, there have been numerous cases of assaults, thefts, sexual offences, defalcation of monies, drunkenness, chronic absenteeism, attempts at molestation of patients or their relatives and many similar acts. The management in past years have not been able to effectively control these matters of indiscipline for the simple reason that the Unions have obstructed every single attempt at maintaining discipline.

The most recent example of this is the present strike which has been called for the single purpose of obstructing the normal process of an enquiry to look into acts of violence and intimidation.

No organisation, particularly a social organisation, can ever hope to carry out its obligations to the public and to the nation, if its management is obstructed from maintaining discipline by continued acts of terrorism and violence in order that indiscipline may flourish.

I have given you this long introduction with the intention of explaining to you the strong spirit that prevails among the 2,000 loyal workers of the Christian Medical College and Hospital. These loyal staff have paid a very heavy price in terms of receiving abuses and insults, particularly young ladies such as nurses and clerks, attempts at disrobing them at public, assaults, violence, smearing of clothes with human excreta and many other acts which are not acceptable in a civilized society. They have taken courage from the fact that the management has at last made a very strong attempt at putting down such uncivilised acts in future by terminating the services of the most prominent of the ring leaders of the groups that have caused such terrorism and violence. Therefore, they have been and will continue to be strongly supportive of the management in its attempts to root out these evil elements which have beset the hospital. So much about the attitude of the staff.

There is another angle which I must very seriously bring to your notice. It is simply this. If these 15 people whose acts of indiscipline which surpass all other acts are to be reemployed under your guarantees, then by the same token over 15-20 other employees who have been terminated over the past seven or eight years for much lesser offences will also expect to be reinstated, possibly under such guarantees from friends such as yourselves. There would also be an expectation that the five who have been found guilty of corruption with the M.B.B.S. selections may also have this expectation for reinstatement, also under similar guarantees. By the same token, in future for every offence committed, kind hearted friends like you may possibly come up with fresh assurances. This would give a suggestion or idea to staff that they enjoy a degree of freedom to commit acts of indiscipline with the knowledge that when they are in difficulties or when their services are terminated, they will obtain the services of friends like you to have them re-employed.

All this means only one thing, that the management will become totally ineffective in maintaining discipline. True, in your generosity and your kindness to these 15 terminated employees you are prepared to give assurances and guarantees, both legal and otherwise, on behalf of the 15 terminated people. Is it right on the part of the management to expect that all the other employees will maintain standards of discipline such as is necessary to run the hospital, when they know that guarantees can be furnished when they are found guilty of misconduct? Sirs, as a representative of the management, 1 feel that your kind gesture on behalf of the 15 terminated employees may help the management at the present situation, but at a future date which may be quite soon, the management may involve itself into great difficulties and we may not only relapse into the state of terrorism that was prevalent earlier, but even into a worse state.

I trust now I have stated the problems peculiar to the management as I have stated the point of view of the vast majority of loyal staff.

To come to the third point, namely, the legality of the guarantees which you so kindly offer: you will recall that I promised to check your request with two of our legal advisers, whose reputation and standing in the legal profession is well known throughout this country. I have the highest regard for them, inasmuch as they have a high admiration for this institution. They have given a very considered and impartial legal opinion, again in the very best interests of this institution. We have checked with them independently and therefore, one is not aware of what the other has said. In their independent opinion, whatever legal guarantees are given by whichever eminent person, such legal guarantees only highlight the deep concern of eminent personalities in the welfare of the person or persons for whom the guarantee is given, but will not be valid in a court of law, as ground for proceeding against indisciplined employees at a future date.

Therefore, while deeply appreciating your generous offer to guarantee on behalf of the 15 terminated employees, it still does not help us in any way, if these terminated employees continue to misbehave.

Therefore, on all these three grounds, my colleagues, both in administration and in the institution, and I very respectfully and yet regretfully say that your kind offer may not be accepted.

Once again, we join together in offering you our humble regards and gratitude for all that you have done for us and which we are confident you will continue to do for us.

You may justifiably ask what is the future of the hospital, particularly when pressures are mounting. As you well know, many of us are in this institution because we have dedicated our future not only to the service of suffering people, but also to the service of a divine Creator, to whom we belong. Therefore, when this deep dedication to a divine power governs the thoughts, actions and feelings of the vast majority of people, I sense the courage and the faith that whatever will befall the Christian Medical College and Hospital we shall carry on the responsibilities which we are required to fulfil. In this process, there may be many difficulties, enhanced physical violence, imprisonment, further insults and abuses, institutional taxations and fines, and many other things which I cannot possibly conceive of, but which are yet within the realms of possibility. However, the spirit of the Christian Medical College and Hospital, a spirit which was kindled by the spirit of its Founder, Dr Ida S. Scudder, which in turn is a spark from the divine Spirit, refused to be crushed whatever the difficulties. I am sure many, many here among the staff will cheerfully shed our blood or undergo any difficulties or privations without any thought for self with the single thought that in these difficulties we are serving our patients and our Creator.

There is also one other confidence we have that the spirit of friendship and affection which you have so visibly demonstrated to us will yet abide with us and that you will continue to sustain us in our adversities, as you have done in the past. I may assure you, Sirs, that efforts are still being made at various other levels to come to an understanding with those who are on strike and with the rest of us. The solutions are not easy, particularly when very important principles are involved. There are moves to call into conference the Governing Council at a much earlier date than previously scheduled, so that they may also give us a sense of direction, policy and purpose, and perhaps find a way out of this deadlock. The Council was scheduled to meet towards the end of next month, but there are several Council members who are now anxious to bring it forward, so that further considerations of the present problem may take place.

Once again, please accept the humble gratitude of all of us here, doctors and nurses, technicians and other staff, the management and I, for all that you have done for us and for all the help that you will give us in our days of difficulty. With all good wishes and prayers.

Yours very sincerely,

(Sd.) L. B. M. Joseph

The involvement of the three dissident senior Faculty in the strike directly resulted in the State Government taking a position against the Institution, insisting that all the disciplinary action taken thus far should be rescinded and all the terminated employees should be reinstated. The Administration and the Loyal staff including the Faculty were clear that there could be no compromise on the issue of corruption and indiscipline. A group of Senior citizens of Vellore formed a 'Save CMC' committee in support of the Institutions stand. The citizens of Vellore were concerned about the economic impact on the town of the decreasing number of patients visiting Vellore. Several of them made discreet enquiries of the Faculty of what were the contingency plans and were told that even if it meant shifting the Institution elsewhere, there was no question of yielding on the issue of discipline. Rumours began to circulate in town about an invitation to shift CMC to Hyderabad and the attitude towards the striking workers subtly changed with any sympathy felt towards them gradually decreasing..

The Government meanwhile increased the pressure on the administration so that they would agree to the withdrawal of the disciplinary action on Alpheus and the other workers. The Chairman was brought by car from Madurai by the Government. The Collector was his old student. He arranged for his stay in the Government guest house in town and requested him to persuade the administration to reinstate all the dismissed employees. However the administration, the faculty and staff were clear that such action would foster indiscipline and destroy the Institution and that they would not agree to it. The faculty were threatened with severe consequences if they did not change their stance but they were clear that they were not be prepared for any compromise with corrupt and indisciplined colleagues. After two days at Vellore the Government took him back home as they realised he was on a failed mission in which he was not interested! It was clear that the Chairman shared the views of the Faculty on maintenance of discipline.

On the 10th of March there were strong indications that the Director Dr. LBM Joseph was likely to be arrested. He was at home that day and when the legal advisors in Madras were contacted they wanted that he should immediately proceed to Madras and file for anticipatory bail in the Madras High Court. LBM with Dr. VI Mathan as his driver left for Madras after a quick early lunch. They took a route avoiding the highway and reached the Office of the Legal Advisors about half an hour before closure of the High Court. All papers for Anticipatory Bail were signed and submitted before the Court closed but the actual Bail papers would be available only the next day. We were advised that we should ensure that there were no arrests that night and actually had to change our place of residence thrice during the night. The anticipatory bail orders were received by lunch time and we started back to Vellore the next day.

Meanwhile high drama was happening in Vellore. Shortly before lunch the police came to arrest the Director from the Hospital campus. They found Professor KV Mathai, a nationally recognised Neurosurgeon and Associate Director as the Acting Director for the day and arrested him and took him to the Police Office in the Fort. In fact the Collector and the Police soon recognised that they had made a tactical error. Many of the shops in town downed their shutters to protest the arrest. As there was unrest in the town the Police who had formally arrested Dr. Mathai requested him to go back to the Hospital. He refused to leave without proper bail being granted to him. He had to be kept overnight in the Office of the Superintendent of Police so that the District Magistrate could grant him bail the next day! Dr. Mathai was well known in the country with many of his patients in high positions in the Central Government. The news of his arrest spread widely and the high handed action of the Police was condemned by many. This arrest persuaded the Central Government that the time had come for them to intervene in the situation.

The then Central Home Minister, came to Madras and held discussions with the State Chief Minister and with the CMC Administration. The stand taken by CMC was recognised by the

Central Government as correct and they persuaded the State Government to announce the withdrawal of the strike on the floor of the State Assembly on Saturday March 15th without CMCH announcing any concession to the strikers. The Chief Minister announced that CMC had an adamant and stubborn administration and that he was providing alternate employment for all the terminated employees and advised the workers of CMC to join duty. The Institution started to function with the appearance of normality from Monday March 17, 1975. The Seventy day Strike was over. It was clearly a victory for the administration and the loyal staff! The concluding paragraphs of the Directors report to the May 1975 meeting of the Council is quoted below

"Council will realise that this tragic period through which we are passing is largely the result of the activities of a small group of dissident staff who, for their own ends, have introduced political influences into the life of the Organisation, have persistently opposed the administration and have attempted to subvert the authority of the Executive and Council. In the past there have been attempts at reconciliation, but recent events have unfortunately shown that there is an. unbridgeable gap between these elements and the rest of the Institution. My colleagues in the Administration and I are regretfully convinced that the time has come when it is impossible to effectively carry out the work of the Institution while these elements continue to subvert its life. We therefore have no alternative but to recommend to this Council that ·appropriate action be taken immediately in order to save the Institution."

The Council considered the detailed reports of the Director to the Council, during and after the strike and at their meeting in October 1975 unanimously decided to terminate the services of the three senior faculty who sat on hunger strike at the end of January. (Cl: 4637: 10-75). This ended the saga of the seventy day strike officially but the end of the legal problems that started with the admission corruption finally was given a quietus only in 1989 when the Honourable Supreme Court of India appointed Mr Justice Natarajan (retired Supreme Court Judge) as an Arbitrator to finally solve the dispute with the employees terminated during the strike. Why did the issue take so long to resolve?

In 1975 when the strike and related problems started the Institution was considered as an educational Institution and the provisions of the Industrial Disputes Act (ID Act) were not applicable to educational Institutions. Hence there was no possibility of raising a labour dispute under the ID act. However in 1976 the judgement in a case known as the 'Bangalore Water and Sewerage Board Dispute" changed the very definition of Industry and Hospitals and Educational Institutions became subject to the ID act. Soon after this the Labour union who had spearheaded the seventy day strike raised an industrial dispute regarding the employees whose services were terminated on January 8 1975. The Institution fought this ID from the Vellore Labour court to the labour Tribunal and the High Court in Madras and finally to the Honourable Supreme Court. In each level it became clear that while the stand of the Institution was morally correct and the services of these employees had to be terminated in the best interest of the patients who depended on the institution the strict provisions of the Industrial Disputes Act had been violated by this action. How could this dilemma be resolved?

The Hon. Supreme Court appointed Mr. Justice (Retired) Natarajan, a former Judge of the Hon. Supreme Court, as an Arbitrator whose award would be binding on all parties. After detailed hearings of all parties and recording evidence the Honourable Arbitrator came to the conclusion that while the Industrial Disputes act was applicable to Hospitals there was a unique feature that had to be considered. In factories and commercial establishment there are only two parties, Management and Labour to any dispute. The product of their cooperative activity are commercial products and a dispute leading to a strike or other industrial action does not directly threaten lives. However In any dispute in a Hospital environment there is a vital group whose interests must be paramount. These are the patients who approach a Hospital for life sustaining help and any industrial action that puts at risk the life of patients would be completely unacceptable. He therefore concluded that the management of a hospital cannot be compelled to continue in employment any employee in whom they had lost confidence. Such continuance of employment would mean that the management was forced to put the life and wellbeing of patients who come to them under employees in whom they had no confidence. He enunciated that in such instances it would be justified to monetarily compensate such employees rather than reinstate them in positions where they would be responsible for the life of patients. Suitable compensation was worked out by the Arbitrator and finally the Industrial dispute that started in 1976 was put to rest in1989, fourteen years later.

What are the lessons to be learnt from this very traumatic period in the life of the Institution? We learnt that the maintenance of discipline is primary to the life and welfare of the patients who come to a Hospital. It is essential that all who work for patients recognise their primary responsibility to maintain the discipline of the Institution. Any compromise either by the management or the workers will inevitably lead to problems. A heavy price has to be paid to recover from such situations. The management of CMCV was not vigilant in the maintanence of discipline during the early seventies and the price of that was the strike. Dr LBM Joseph with his commitment to Christ and his clear understanding that CMCV was His Institution offered the leadership to guide out of the crisis. The crisis also showed that it was essential to be loyal to the Institution. It was the desire to promote themselves that guided the leaders of the strike to take this destructive path.

There has been industrial peace at CMCV for the last forty five years since the strike. The Institution has grown many times in size since then but the strategies of discussion at all level starting from Unit and Departmental Committees, The General Service Board, The Medical and Nursing Service Boards and representation of the General Service Board on the Governing Council have contributed to this stability. This model of participatory management should be sustained to ensure healthy working of the Institution for many more decades.

Chapter 10

Recovery and Rebuilding 1975 to 1986

Dr LBM Joseph

The seventy day strike ended by the middle of March 1975 and the Institution started on the task of recovery and rebuilding. The first priority of the Administration was to improve communication with the staff and Faculty. Each unit and Department was encouraged to start regular meetings where all staff would jointly consider future developmental plans and also address issues of concern to the work or life of the Department and Institution. Copies of the minutes of these meetings were given to the concerned administrative Officers who made sure that follow up action was taken as required. Staff thus had a channel through which their concerns and suggestions were brought to the attention of the Administration. The Administrative Officers and the Heads of Departments and Units made sure that all follow up action was communicated to the staff. Elections were held in all departments and Units to select representatives of the Class III or IV staff to form the General Service Board, chaired by the General Superintendent.

The General Services Board met regularly, usually at monthly intervals to discuss issues of concern. All Administrative Officers usually participated in the meetings of the General Services Board so that issues raised by the staff could be promptly addressed. The effective functioning of this system gave a sense of ownership and participatory management to the staff, thus improving the spirit and atmosphere of the institution.

The leadership team consisted of Dr. LBM Joseph, Professor of Surgery as Director; Dr. KV Mathai Professor of Neurosurgery as Associate Director, Dr. CK Job, Professor of Pathology, Principal, Dr. Jacob Abraham, Professor of Neurosurgery, Medical Superintendent, Dr. M Mohan Rao, Professor of Urology, General Superintendent, Miss A Kuruvilla, Professor of Nursing, Dean College of Nursing, Miss Alice Jane David, Professor of Nursing, Nursing Superintendent and Mr CC Jacob, Treasurer. Administrative officers had small teams, usually from the faculty, who shared their responsibilities as Associates or Deputies. In this way many of the Faculty gained administrative experience and provided a pool from which new leaders could be selected when the term of any Administrative Officer was completed. Normally only the Treasurer and the General Superintendent would be considered for further terms after the first term of service, which at this time was seven years. As patients flocked to Vellore and the work load increased it became clear that the Director, Treasurer and the General Superintendent should be full time responsibilities.

Mohan Rao, an excellent urologist who did the first Renal Transplant in India at Vellore, was also the General Superintendent responsible for maintaining discipline in the Institution. Several clerical and attender level employees who tried to restart activities they had indulged in prior to the Seventy Day strike were pulled up and some were discharged from service after due process. There was considerable anger towards the General Superintendent from a vocal section of the staff because of these actions. Regrettably Mohan decided to resign from the Institution and migrate to Australia. This was a loss to the Institution not only of a good administrator but also of the leading urologist of the country. He continued as a good friend of the Institution and was active in the Friends of Vellore in Australia. Fortunately he had trained his colleague Dr. Pandey well and Mohan's departure did not significantly impact the renal transplant program. Dr. PSS Sundar Rao, Professor of Bio-Statistics took over as the General Superintendent in 1977.

The Planning Cell was reactivated by the Director soon after the strike was over. A detailed report on the strategy for the next five years, prepared by the Planning Cell with significant inputs by the staff, was accepted by the Council as the framework for further development. The Council also approved the Staff Service Rules (Cl: 4721:6-76) as well as a policy regarding Core Research Staff (Cl:4722:6-76). This policy on Core Research Staff and the decision to reserve up to one third of one percent of the Maintenance Budget to support research activities were significant decisions which strengthened research in the Institution. Faculty interested in developing research could get seed grants from the Institution's research funds to develop their ideas to the point where they had preliminary findings with which they could compete for substantial external research grants.

Scholarships were provided to support the education of the children of lower paid staff in the Institution. These scholarships made it possible for the children of many staff to study in the Ida Scudder School. Ten percent of the seats in the Medical College and other educational programs were made available for staff children if they had the requisite academic credentials. All staff children could compete for admission to all academic programs. The selection was based only on academic merit of the children decided at the entrance test without any consideration of the job title of the parent. At the selection committees, after a decision on the number of seats that would be set aside for staff children was made for each course, an anonymous list of eligible candidates ranked in order of their academic merit would be presented identified only by the registration number and the requisite number selected based on their marks. The code would be broken only after completion of selection to identify the children. Of course faculty whose children were competing for admission were not part of the selection process for that year. The record shows that in several instances children of attenders were admitted to the MBBS program on merit while the children of Administrators or senior Faculty did not make the grade in the competitive process.

The institution held an International Consultation in which, in addition to the administration and representation of the senior faculty, there was external experts both from India and from abroad. After a careful study and discussion of all aspects of the work and life of the institution,the Consultation unanimously adopted the following report.

1. This consultation was called in view of several factors among which the following may be mentioned: ·

    (a) We are in the midst of a transition from a society which was willing to accept leadership from a trained elite, to a society which insists on the full participation of the common man.

b) As a corollary of this, there has come a new direction in medical thinking, frequently sponsored by W.H.O. and W.C.C. and other organisations, which places the emphasis upon the health of the entire community rather than upon the availability of curative facilities for a minority.

(c) The growing awareness of the increasing costs of running this institution and the severe limitations on available income, as has been highlighted in the Prahalad report.

2. The Consultation reaffirms the validity of the objectives as stated in the Memorandum of the Association. Within the framework of these objectives, the institution has developed a variety of forms of training for service and leadership in the health work of the nation in accordance with the changing needs and opportunities of the times. The factors mentioned in the first paragraph challenge us to consider how the institution can pioneer in the coming decade.

3. This Consultation is led to affirm that the Christian Medical College is called to pioneer in the application of the new concept of total community health to every aspect of its work in training, research and service.

4.   We believe that Christian Medical College is uniquely placed to pioneer in this matter for two reasons: (i) because of the standing of the Institution in the medical world; (ii) because through the churches which make up the Association, the

Christian Medical College can reach out into the whole community through the widespread network of Christian hospitals and through the still more widespread network of the congregations in towns and villages.

5. We recommend that the Institution: (a) explore ways of reorienting the training of medical, nursing and para-medical students so that they may be able effectively to fit into the health team needed for community care; (b) develop research of the highest calibre into the many problems of community health; (c) investigate the desirability of training other cadres of health workers.

6. This Consultation, representing both the Christian Medical College Administration and the supporting bodies, would like to ask the churches whether they would welcome help from the Christian Medical College in terms of training, advice and guidance in reorienting their medical programmes towards a total community approach, and preparing members of the congregations for participation in the healing ministry. If the response from the churches is positive, then the churches will be obligated to help the Christian Medical College to find resources from outside to subsidise this project.

7. While emphasising the role of community medicine, we reaffirm the importance of the present training and service in the specialities and of the research programmes. We also recognise that the Institution may be led to develop other areas of specialisation and research. In planning future development it is desirable that there be consultations with comparable institutions in India, government and other agencies.

8. The Consultation urges the Administration to continue to explore ways and means of reducing the potential gap between income and expenditure and of raising endowment. We also wish to bring to the notice of the supporting bodies the fact that each medical student costs the institution Rs 60,000 for the first five and a half years of training (the student pays Rs 720 per year) and during the last financial year about Rs 20 lakhs was spent on free treatment. We request the supporting bodies to study the implications of this.

The Consultation recorded its gratitude to all the Church leaders who were present and in particular to Mr JC. McGilvray, Executive Director, Christian Medical Commission of the World Council of Churches and Dr Martin Scheel, Executive Director of the German Medical Mission, Tubingen, for their participation in the proceedings of the Consultation.

Several senior professors retired on attaining the age of superannuation or took voluntary retirement after twenty five years of service in 1976. This included Prof. HS Bhatt, pioneering Urologist and the first Surgical postgraduate from the Institution, Prof. Mrs Prema Bhat, Professor of Microbiology, Prof. C Bhatktaviziam, Head Department of Dermatology, and Prof Arnold Desmond, Head Department of ENT.

Prof Arnold Desmond, a graduate and postgraduate from the Madras Medical College joined Ear Nose and Throat (ENT) Department of CMCV in 1947. He was an excellent surgeon who also had skills in civil engineering which he used to good effect in assisting the extensive construction activities on the developing campus. His contributions to the planning of the Outpatient block and the Men Internes Quarters were particularly noteworthy.

He wrote an autobiographic book titled "Years Of Fame" describing his work in CMCV as the Institution was developing from 1951 to 1974 which also summarised the earlier years. His contributions to construction on the campuses are documented along with how he developed the ENT department. He is a good example of the commitment of graduates from other Institutions making significant contributions to the growth and development of CMCV.

At the end of the 1960's a UK based Trust informed the Institution that they were interested to provide funds for a major innovative health thrust in a rural community near Vellore. It was decided that this program should have a leader with a vision to develop a community health program with a major focus on social development. Although these funds were available from the end of the sixties the Director and others searched for such a leader for nearly six years. Dalip Mukherjee, a CMC Graduate who had specialised in Tropical Public Health and Health Economics in UK, visited Vellore in 1975.   LBM challenged him with this new initiative and Dalip took up the challenge to develop a Rural Unit for Health and Social Action (RUHSA) in the KV Kuppam Block. The Institution already had a small community based health program in that block, located about fifteen kilo meters to the Northwest of Vellore which formed the nucleus of this new initiative.

At about the same time Abraham Joseph, a Vellore graduates who inherited the leadership of the Community Health Department of the College from Drs KG Koshy and V Benjamin decided that the focus of the program in the Kaniambady Block, to the south of the College campus, where they had been working for over two decades, should increasingly be on development.

The name of the Department, already changed from Preventive and Social Medicine to Community Health was further modified to Community Health and Development (CHAD). Thus two different strategies for health and development were to be tried out by the Institution. In RUHSA social action would be the route to transform the health of the community while in CHAD improving health was the base that facilitated social and economic development.

It is not proposed to compare, contrast and evaluate the development and progress of these two strategies, both of which are now successful, large, nationally and internationally recognised public health programs. Their developmental history and contributions to medical education and community development and health, deserve detailed documentation. The Institution learned from these two innovative attempts that clear goals and effective leadership are the key to success. Both CHAD and RUHSA have significantly improved the health and social indices of the communities they served, irrespective of the strategies followed! However one of the original objectives, wide participation by all Faculty of the Institution in Community Health activities, did not really materialise, as every member of the Faculty was deeply involved in making their department the best in the country! The other objective was the reproducibility of these programs in other community development blocks. Unfortunately these programs depended so much on the initiative of the leader as well as the significant financial inputs that while they produced excellent results in the community that was served, they were not easily reproducible.

Important policies and strategies were developed and applied during the latter half of the seventies. The staff Service

Rules were codified (Cl:4721:6-76) and printed booklets were made available to all departments and staff. The policy regarding Faculty who would primarily be involved in research (Core Research Staff, Cl:4722:6-76) was clearly defined and became a major impetus to the development of research at Vellore. This important resolution is quoted in full below:

Cl:4722:6-76

"Resolved:

(1)to affirm the commitment of the management to a continued presence and emphasis on research as well as teaching and service in the institution, and to plan to include a cadre of research workers as an integral part of the institution and staff. At the same time it is evident that the maintenance budget already in deficit due to the costs of education, with the main source of income coming from patients' fees, cannot possibly absorb such an expense. It is therefore further resolved that initially a small group of senior staff who are presently involved In research be taken on to institutional support, their salaries to come from the interests of the research endowment fund, with the expectation that these investigators, should existing project funding cease, would be able to generate project support for other research staff. Subsequently, we hope that as the endowment fund enlarges, a greater degree of support of both staff and research work may be permissible from this fund.

(2) to request the Executive Committee to examine the possibility of allotting 1/3rd of 1 percent from maintenance budget for research and report back to Council.

Based on this resolution one third of one per cent of the annual maintenance budget was made available for the support of research initiatives by the faculty. This policy allowed several large and multidisciplinary research groups to develop. Several of the research projects initially funded by competitive grants from external agencies, mainly from governmental agencies, grew and became large clinical research programs. When the external grants term was over, the problem was how to offer continuity of service to the trained and skilled scientists and technologists whose salaries were from external grants. The Principal Investigators in many instances obtained competitive external grants to continue research, but the possibility of Institutional support ensured that key scientists were able to work with the knowledge that they would not have to worry about continuity of support for their salaries. The Enterovirus research group, the Neurosciences research group and the Wellcome research group are examples of such initially externally funded major projects which evolved into permanent primarily research Units with a strong clinical connection. The strong clinical connection ensured continuity with departmental and Institutional funds in several of these instances. The Institutional policies facilitated the coming together of multidisciplinary skills to develop most of these research groups.

Young faculty with children growing up, who were resident on two separate campuses, presented challenges that had to be resolved such as transportation between the College and the Hospital especially for clinicians to attend emergency calls and good education for staff children. The salaries at Vellore in the sixties, even with free housing did not permit saving enough for the purchase of a personal car unless there were personal financial resources. The cost of a car (only two models were available then, the Fiat and the Ambassador) was about the same as the annual salary of a Professor at Vellore! In 1970 none of the Indian faculty, already the majority of the staff, had cars. Realising the importance of good communication between the two campuses the Institution provided a telephone system which connected the two campuses through the town telephone exchange, with individual phones in each ward, office and in all faculty houses. In this pre-mobile phone era the internal telephone system connecting all clinical facilities, offices and residences on both the campuses facilitated good clinical work. Frequent official transport by Institutional vehicles was provided directly between the two campuses, with stopovers at the Schell Eye campus when needed. These operated at fixed times and many clinicians felt that it did not offer sufficient flexibility to them. Transport was also available on request for emergencies. The obvious long term answer was cars for individual faculty. The problem solved itself as all faculty were encouraged to go abroad for up to three years for further training (study leave), soon after their confirmation. Most of them managed to save enough to purchase a car on their return! The Institution provided a reasonable transport allowance on a reimbursable basis.

As faculty children grew up, finding good schools for them in and around Vellore became a challenge. Nursery schools were started on both the Hospital and College campuses and a Primary School on the College campus. These schools were operated by societies formed by the Faculty and staff in space provided by the Institution. Officially these school were not part of the Institution. The Nursery Schools catered to the children of staff resident on the particular campus. Admission to the primary school, the Vidyalayam on the College Campus, was exclusively for children of staff. A sliding scale of fees was fixed, according to the salary of the parents, to make it affordable for the children of lower paid staff. School buses were arranged to take the children of staff resident on the Hospital campus, picking up children of staff resident in the town on the way. The Vidyalayam provided an opportunity for several staff wives who were trained teachers to utilise the skills they had been trained for. Mrs Betty Baker the wife of Prof Selwyn Baker was the first Principal and she was followed by Mrs Susan Abraham, a trained and experienced teacher, the wife of Prof Jacob Abraham, Professor of Neurosurgery.

Several members of the staff in association with friends from the town then started a full K to 12 School on land that the Hospital had in Viruthampatt, just north of the Palar Bridge, about two kilometres from the Hospital. This Ida Scudder School has proven invaluable to the welfare of staff families of CMCV. Generations of staff children and others from the town have been given good education, a major factor in retaining good Faculty in the Institution. Scholarships are provided to children of lower paid staff to ensure that they can study at Scudder School. In fact several children of the lower paid employees of CMCV have completed Medicine and Nursing at CMCV primarily as a result of their training at Scudder School. Neither Vidyalayam nor Scudder School are officially part of the Institution, although Vidyalayam is on the college campus and Scudder School on land belonging to CMCV. They are run by independent societies, all the members belonging to CMCV staff in the case of Vidyalayam, while the Scudder School Association has members from the Town also. These two educational Institutions are excellent examples of the contribution of the Institution to life in Vellore.

The atmosphere in the Institution was peaceful during this period and there was no effort by external forces to try and revive the Union. Several months after his termination Alpheus got a stay of the termination order from the local Munsiff's Court and had to be temporarily reinstated. After a lengthy legal battle which went up to the Madras High Court the services of Alpheus Joseph were finally terminated, as the Courts upheld the disciplinary action on him. The architect of the Union and the strike, Jayakaran Joseph, did not return to the Institution at the end of the study leave granted to him. The Council recorded after due process that Jayakaran had abandoned services (Cl 4902:3-77) thereby closing a turbulent chapter.

The disputes raised by the Labour Union regarding the employees terminated at the beginning of the strike ultimately reached the Honourable Supreme Court of India. After several hearings the Court referred this dispute to arbitration by a retired Judge of the Hon. Supreme Court in 1989. The Arbitrator after a series of hearings held that the termination of the employees at the beginning of the seventy day strike was on valid grounds, as It was the result of loss of confidence in them by the management because of their acts of indiscipline. However this was done without the necessary due process according to the dictates of the Industrial Dispute(ID) Act and therefore they were legally eligible for reinstatement. Hospitals even Teaching Hospitals like CMCV come under the definition of Industry in the Act and the provision of the ID Act would have to be strictly applied. The Arbitrator however held that unlike in the usual industrial situation, in a Hospital it was essential that the Management had absolute confidence in all their employees as they were dealing with the life of individual patients and not inanimate industrial production. Lives of Patients would be vulnerable if the management was forced to place their care in the hands of employees in whom they had lost confidence. Therefore in the circumstances the Arbitrator awarded financial compensation for all the terminated employees and did not order their reinstatement. This was accepted by all and there has been no attempt to revive the Union or their disruptive activities since then. The crucial role of the confidence of the management in all staff in a hospital is an important policy guideline for labour relationship in patient care situations.

The faculty after their experience during the strike took a more proactive role in the Institution. It was recognised that even though it was one of the largest Medical educational complexes in the country, it would be unlikely that senior administrators could be recruited from outside because the salary and emoluments were not competitive with other private institutions of comparable size or to what they could earn in private practice. Furthermore such external recruits may not fully subscribe to the Institutional ethos. The motivating factor for the vast majority of the Faculty to continue to work at CMCV was the ability to provide Health care of the highest professional quality in the spirit of Christ. This ensured a mostly Christian senior staff, with a commitment to service and willingness to accept financial rewards significantly lower than what they could get elsewhere. However they were more than compensated by the Christian and professional atmosphere they worked in. Several undergraduates and Postgraduates of Vellore who were not nominally Christian subscribed fully to the ethos and continue to give a life time of service at Vellore. They have contributed richly to the spirit of the Institution. This unity in diversity is a hallmark of CMCV. The two campuses are excellent residential facilities and campus life with the students is particularly rewarding.

In the aftermath of the strike the Director initiated discussions with the Faculty to define the way forward. The result of extensive discussions the Director held with the Faculty subsequent to the strike was "A statement on the priorities of CMC for the next 5 years". This document was presented to and accepted by the Council in 1978 by a resolution that stated in part:

" It was suggested that a final paragraph should be added to emphasize that this is a Christian College with Christian interest and Christian concern for all needy and suffering. The mainspring of the excellence of the institution is the Christian commitment of all it's staff. In all these efforts CMC will ever bear in mind its responsibility to bear witness to Christ's concern for the poor and downtrodden and for the total welfare of man."

Various developments have occurred in this institution not necessarily because of planning but because of the enthusiasm and hard work of some people. The spirit of Christ had been instrumental for making people develop specialities and bring about new developments. This has been the main distinction between CMC and other medical colleges.

To make continuous efforts to provide the most modern facilities in every department and speciality in accordance with the requirements of the Nation."

The Council,while emphasising and reiterating the Christian character of the Institution and the key role played by the Faculty and staff, highlighted the need for the Institution to be at the cutting edge of health care technology to serve India, while maintaining its essential Christian nature. The commitment of the faculty and staff was to provide the highest quality of health care to all who visited Vellore as patients and also to the adjacent communities they served. The mandate for training and research were integral to excellence of service. It was accepted by all the faculty that service in the name of Christ has to be of the highest quality and should be available to all who sought it. The problem was the increasing technological nature of the service and its increasing cost. There was also some confusion in the minds of many friends regarding the relative roles of primary care and specialised technology in the life and ministry of Christian Institutions. In contrast to those who believed that primary care should be the main, if not the sole, means of witnessing especially through service to the poorest of the poor, the Institution witnessed through the best available health care technology adapted to serve the needs of its neighbouring communities and the thousands from all over India who came to Vellore for help.

The mixture of primary care and high technology which characterised the Vellore approach to the Healing Ministry was explored at length in an International Consultation at Vellore in 1980 and the 'Both /And' philosophy that guided the witness of the Institution was formalised. Vellore offers a unique opportunity for people of different faiths to work together harmoniously to witness effectively in Christ's Healing Ministry. As long as you are an effective partner in the work of Christs healing ministry and willing to work harmoniously to care for the sick and train students, your particular theological beliefs are accepted as your personal conviction. At Vellore there is hardly any effort to proselytise personal interpretations of Theology.

At this time there was an effort to present the work of the Institution to the Christian Health Commission of the World Council of Churches (WCC) headquartered in Geneva, Switzerland. This was with the hope that significant financial help would be provided through the Commission to augment the charity work of the Institution and offset the very large educational subsidy for training MBBS students. The WCC however subscribed unreservedly to the view that primary care was the best and possibly the only way to witness in the Healing ministry and was not willing to accept the Vellore philosophy that cutting edge technological health care was also an essential part of such witness. This difference of perspective toward the healing ministry has been to the mutual disadvantage of both organisations. It has meant that the resources and expertise of the two largest Christian organisations in the healing ministry have not worked together to maximise their impact.

LBM Joseph was appointed as the Director in 1974 and when his seven year term ended in 1981 the Council extended his appointment for a second term as Director. He had offered outstanding leadership during the 1975 strike and was the main driver of the recovery, but several senior staff had reservations about his continuation for a second term. Was he the right person to lead the Institution into the future which was turning out to be technology driven? The commitment of the Institution to technology was signalled by the renal transplant program started in 1974 and the commissioning of the Betatron for the treatment of cancer patients in 1978. All departments were encouraged to offer the best of their speciality at Vellore, while maximising their charity work with the philosophy that none who came to Vellore should be denied medical help on financial grounds. The annual budget of the Institution each year showed large deficits but by the end of the financial year the deficit would be largely covered by the additional earnings through the year. This was a difficult balancing act but the staff and the administration proved adequate to the task.

The faculty paid a financial price for this balancing act. The salaries and emoluments of the non- medical staff were comparable to what they would earn in state government service or in private sector, especially when the free medical benefits for the families were factored in. However, the faculty salaries were substantially lower than what they could earn even in government service let alone private practice. The strength of the Institution has been the Faculty committed to the philosophy of the Institution who unreservedly give a lifetime of service. Earnings during the three years of study leave all faculty were eligible for soon after confirmation and sabbatical leave later during their career, usually compensated for the low salaries to a great extent. Hardly any confirmed Faculty resigned due to a feeling of insufficient salary. During the last nearly sixty years the Faculty has become Indian and none who stayed on suffered significant financial difficulties.

At the time of superannuation at the age of sixty, after at least fifteen years of confirmed service, all were eligible for statutorily required Provident Fund and Gratuity payments. These were lump sum payments which if wisely invested could provide a very modest monthly income. The retired staff and spouse were also eligible for free medical care at Vellore for the rest of their lives. However for many staff these amounts received on superannuation were barely enough to settle the debts incurred during their years of service especially for children's education and marriage. The resignation of two senior faculty several years prior to superannuation, in the latter half of the seventies, challenged Dr LBM. These two faculty who were close personal friends of LBM made it very clear that the reasons they were resigning and going in for practice was their fear that they would not be able to provide for their children on Vellore salaries and they were worried about what would happen after their superannuation. These resignations prompted LBM with the Treasurer Mr. CC Jacob to devise the 'CMC Vellore Special Superannuation Scheme for long service'. This was in addition to the statutorily mandated Provident Fund and Gratuity benefits already available. The scheme was extended to cover all confirmed staff who had superannuated at the age of sixty or later if they were still alive, even if they retired prior to the initiation of the scheme.

Currently the superannuation benefits on retiring at the age of sixty after completing a minimum of fifteen years of continuous service after confirmation consists of contributory Provident Fund and Gratuity payment, as well as the Special Superannuation Scheme. The first two are statutorily mandated lump sum payments and Government rules guide the payment. Careful investment of the amounts received as Provident Fund and Gratuity can ensure a regular modest income to the retired employee. However for the majority of the employees, especially the lower paid, these payments were primarily a means of settling debts incurred during their working years, particularly for children's education and marriage. It was noticed that many, especially the lower salaried staff were struggling to make ends meet after superannuation and very few were able to invest their provident fund and gratuity to ensure a steady income. In the Special Superannuation Scheme an employee who has thirty years of confirmed service on superannuation at the age of sixty, is eligible for monthly payments of fifty percent of the retirement basic pay and Dearness Allowance as a special superannuation payment. The amount paid is reduced pro-rata if the employee's services is less than thirty years ensuring a minimum of twenty percent of the retirement pay after 15 years of confirmed service. Those with less than fifteen years of service are not eligible for this special scheme meant for individuals who contributed a lifetime of service to Vellore.

There were other important policy decisions during this time. In 1981 it was decided that one third of admissions in all courses should be from the socially and educationally backward sections of society. Since the majority of seats in all educational courses were reserved for candidates sponsored by the supporting Missions and Churches it was necessary to convince them to sponsor children from such backgrounds to all the courses and not just those with right connections. The tradition of one faculty from Vellore being a member of each churches selection committee was a strategy adopted to ensure this social justice. Although this practice has now been in force for over forty years there has been no audit to evaluate its effectiveness. It was also decided that there should not be more than one child from a family in a Medical College class in any one year. Admission to the Medical College is very competitive because of the limited number of seats. The process at Vellore strives to ensure fairness in selection and ensure representation of all churches and supporting bodies while maintaining academic standards. The CMC Hospital is considered equivalent to one of the supporting churches and the children of faculty and staff, who have completed fifteen years of continuous service, are eligible to be sponsored by the Hospital for selection to any of the educational courses. The maximum number of students to be sponsored to any course by a sponsoring body is restricted to ten per cent of the seats, ensuring a fair chance to all.

It was clear by the end of the sixties that the supporting Missions and Churches had limitations as to the finances they could contribute to the maintenance of the Institution. The considerable amounts required for successfully running this very large Health care and educational Institution would of necessity have to be earned. This applied to maintenance as well as capital expenditure. Occasionally large grants could be available for capital needs, but it was clear that significant annual capital expenditure was necessary for the survival of the Institution. Two strategies were adopted to meet this requirement. The Maintenance Budget included a realistic item as depreciation of plant and equipment. This was considered as an expenditure item and at the time of closure of accounts the amount available in this account was transferred to an Equipment Replacement fund, this amount could pay for much of the replacement and upgradation of equipment. A small proportion of the Physicians fees charged to all in patients is set aside as a Development Fund for each clinical department. One third of such amounts generated by the clinical departments is designated to be shared by pre and para clinical departments. This fund is used mainly to purchase new equipment as required to keep up with developments in patient care technology. Each Unit and Department has the provision to maintain a

Departmental special fund to which up to one third of the professional fees charged can be transferred. This fund in addition to purchasing essential equipment, can be used for educational purposes by the staff and for meeting special needs of patients.

The cost of good quality health care is high and the challenge was to provide free or subsidised care to those who needed it but could not afford to pay. The major source of income for the Institution is the fee collected from patients. The fee charged to students is kept low to ensure a reasonable cost of education so that graduates do not have to charge exorbitant fees to their patients to recoup the cost of education. It was realised early that the proportion of free and general ward beds to private ward beds was critical in ensuring the financial wellbeing of the Institution. The Institution charges significantly less than the cost of maintenance of a bed to patients admitted in the general wards. All investigations are also charged to them at standard rates which are cost plus 20 to 50 percent. However Private Ward beds are charged significantly more than cost and higher rates are levied for all investigations. The income thus earned pays for the considerable charity work provided which as per audited statements of accounts each year is around 12 to 15 percent of the total expenditure. About 40 percent of the Outpatients are seen free while about ten percent of inpatients are also treated free of charge. The decision whether a patient is to be a free or subsidised patient is left to the clinician looking after the patient as it was felt that the clinician would be in the best position to judge the ability of the patient to pay.

The finances for capital expenditure are met to a limited extent by the Development Fund and the Equipment Replacement Funds. Individual Departmental special funds also provide significant funds for capital expenditure. The escalating cost of technology meant that significant other resources would have to be found to ensure that the Institution maintained the cutting edge of technology to provide optimum care. The American Schools and Hospitals Abroad (ASHA) program of the Government of the United States of America has played a critical role in fulfilling this need. LBM Joseph's meeting with Senator Mark Hatfield, a key figure in the ASHA program through the Friends of Vellore in 1983 was the beginning of a fruitful association that still continues. Vellore fulfils the three conditions for eligibility for the program, the Institution should have been founded by a US citizen, it should have US citizens continuing on the staff and there should be a US organisation that relates to the developing country recipient institution, through whom appropriate aid could be provided. Over the last four decades the ASHA grants have played a crucial role in ensuring that cutting edge technology is available at Vellore, maintaining it as an Institution of Excellence over the years.

The years of tranquillity that followed the strike in 1975 were utilised to upgrade technology available for patient care. The Institution had gained a reputation for utilisation of technology to improve the care of patients along with excellence of clinical judgement. The major equipment that were acquired during this period included the Betatron for treating cancer patients and a complete gastrointestinal endoscopy set up. The number of patients seeking help at Vellore steadily increased and the finances of the Institution were stable. It was a period of all around growth for the Institution.

Dr. LBM Joseph completed thirteen years as the Director by 1988 and at the request of the Christian Medical college at Ludhiana he was deputed for a year to be a Professor of Surgery there.

Chapter 11

A Period of Growth

Dr. Benjamin M Pulimood

The 1980s marked a period of rapid growth for the Christian Medical College and Hospital, Vellore, while continuing in its core mission of patient care, education and research.

Dr. Benjamin Mani Pulimood, appointed as Director in 1986, was aware that having a motivated team especially the staff was key to achieving the objectives of the Institution. Each development in the history of CMCH had come about as a response to a clear perception of the needs of society from the inception of nursing and medical training in 1909 and 1918; the progressive addition of advanced levels of service and training in various specialties leading to the award of academically higher degrees.

The Wellcome Trust offered to support me and my wife, Dr. Minnie Mathan, as visiting professors for a year from April 1986 in the University of Adelaide and University of Flinders, respectively. This was an opportunity to do full-time research without additional responsibilities of patient care, teaching and administration. This change was enjoyed by us and many new professional contacts were made in Australia.

On my return from the Sabbatical, I continued as Council Secretary and was busy in the Department of Gastroenterology and my research commitments. I was then asked whether I would take on the responsibility of being the Medical Superintendent. I readily agreed because I knew that a well-run hospital was the key to the future of the Institution.

Planning Cell

In a significant move to ensure the progress of the Institution and realising the inefficiency of a large planning cell with all the members of the Administrative Committee and half a dozen senior professors, Dr. Pulimood requested me to find a way for making it more efficient. It was clear that detailed discussions would be needed with all 64 departments, so that staff could articulate their aspirations for future developments. At my request to ensure efficiency of functioning, the Committee was limited to just two people. Dr. AS Kanagasabapathy, Professor of Clinical Biochemistry, and myself. The strategy was that we would act as catalyst to spur the staff of each department to make a clear "Plan of Action" for the future. In one month, we managed to meet every department and to discuss their plans for the next five to ten years and develop a strategy for the future of the Institution. This was then presented for approval to the Council.

However, the problem was the financial cost of this strategy. The Council, after long and careful consideration, approved a loan of eight crores needed for upgradation, to be paid back over ten years. There was considerable opposition to taking a loan as many staff and council members felt that we didn't have the ability to repay the loan. I was able to persuade them using the revenue growth of the Hospital over the preceding four years that this was possible. Thanks to the increased income and the prudence of the treasurer, we had no problem in repaying the loan. This gave a tremendous impetus to the technological development of the Institution and dramatically improved patient care.

At this time, we were fortunate that a linear accelerator for the treatment of cancer patients was gifted by the Asha Programme of the government of the United States of America. This enabled us to treat many more patients with cancer. This made a new venture of radio ablation of deep–seated neurological tumours by a crossbeam technology without open surgery possible. This was the first in India and Southeast Asia and was also used in training doctors from these areas further.

The outpatient facility confined to the first two floors of the building was inadequate to handle the patient services. Fortunately, at this time, Asha building opened and it was possible to transfer the library and all the classrooms to this facility, freeing up the space utilised to improve patient care area. Norman Auditorium, with its valuable conference facilities, continued in the OPD block for larger meetings. The availability of this extra space helped to improve services to the patients.

An entire floor above the radiation therapy department was designed as a Private Patient Service Facility (PPSF), with space for private patient registration, blood collection and waiting area. Rooms were available for consultants to see private patients on prior appointments. This was found to be a major improvement for patients and doctors and facilitated an increase in the number of private patients.

A major change, which facilitated the working of the Hospital was the shift of the casualty and emergency services from the overcrowded out-patient building to the nearby old A ward, which provided more than double the amount of space and other facilities to improve this service. This facility functioned well under Dr. PJ Kuruvilla, who returned from Australia to take charge of it at my request.

Speed and Quality of Service

Recognising the need to enhance both speed and quality of service, computerisation of the Institution was decided upon as a strategic solution. This was not only for patient services but also for the computerisation of entire financial transactions. This system was designed so that there was restricted accessibility of the financial system from the general system of computers.

With this objective in mind, the Institution's technical team approached one of the leading Indian IT service companies who conducted a comprehensive on-site review and assessed existing infrastructure and requirements. Following their evaluation, a detailed report outlining their recommendations for computerisation was submitted. However, the proposed fee far exceeded CMC's budget for this initial phase of the project. This unexpected cost necessitated a re-evaluation of the approach to computerisation.

At this point, Dr. Philip Korula, Professor of Plastic Surgery, offered to develop a programme along with Mr. Chandran, who was in charge of the small computer facility available at that time. The module developed by them for the out–patient investigation services was impressive for its simplicity and the fact that none of the existing investigation forms used in the OPD would have to be changed. CMC was therefore able to develop an in– house programme, which led to the complete computerisation of patient care and financial services. A critical aspect of this network design was the implementation of complete separation between the Hospital's operational systems and the financial data. Two distinct networks were established, ensuring that users with access to the Hospital's general computer system could not access the financial network. This dual–network approach provided a secure and reliable foundation for CMC Vellore's initial foray into computerisation.

There was a significant improvement inpatient service delivery and by streamlining processes, the number of counters patients needed to visit to obtain services was considerably reduced. This innovation resulted in a noticeable decrease in wait times. Furthermore, the introduction of computerised systems facilitated the generation of printouts containing essential information within a matter of seconds. Additionally, networked computers enabled healthcare providers to access patients' reports with greater ease and efficiency. In the context of the early 1990's, these advancements represented a noteworthy accomplishment, marking a significant step forward in leveraging technology to enhance patient care.

The computerisation of certain departments played a critical part during the early 90s period, especially in generating X–rays. The Institution soon developed a completely paperless X–ray system, with the images being stored on the computer. This innovation was the first in the country.

My priority as the Medical Superintendent was to make the Hospital a vibrant, efficient and patient–friendly service facility. The operation theatre was one of the largest areas of the responsibility of the Medical Superintendent. As I was not a surgeon, I had to find an efficient surgeon to run this area.

A careful search convinced me that the most suitable person would be Dr. Ganesh Gopalakrishnan, Professor of Urology, and he discharged this responsibility magnificently.

Dr. C Punnoose Mathew, Professor of Clinical Biochemistry, was appointed as Additional Deputy Medical Superintendent in charge of patient relationships. Punnoose spent at least two hours every day in the morning and evening at the Medical Superintendent's office to meet the patients and solve their problems. This greatly facilitated efficient functioning of the Institution, and actually transformed the image of the Institution in the eyes of the patients. Till then, many patients who came to CMC saw it as a mindless monolith where they had to scramble to get attention. Punnoose facilitated patients' interaction with the Hospital and changed it to a useful and pleasant experience. Medical Superintendent's office soon became the place to which anyone – patient, student or staff – with a problem could come and get a helpful response within 24 hours.

Other Initiatives

1. Mission Activities – Bangalore Baptist Hospital:

    CMC has been involved in helping in the administration of the Bangalore Baptist Hospital, which was started and maintained by the Southern Baptist Convention of the Baptist Church of America. They were concerned that this was a responsibility that they would not be able to discharge permanently. They shared their concerns with the administration. Dr. Pulimood and I decided to try an innovative strategy which could possibly help other struggling hospitals also.

While the land on which the Hospital stood continued to be the property of Southern Baptist Convention, ownership of the Hospital was transferred to the Bangalore Baptist Hospital Society formed by six administrators of CMC by designation, as well as the Director of Bangalore Baptist Hospital. This small group was to administer Bangalore Baptist Hospital similar to the way CMC Council owned and administered by CMC Vellore. An appropriate constitution was drawn up, and a smooth transition was approved by CMC Council. The CMC group visits Bangalore twice a year to approve strategies. The Director of Bangalore Baptist Hospital and a representative selected by the Southern Baptist Convention represent them on the CMC Council. This arrangement has worked successfully with the Institution growing from strength to strength for the last two decades.

2. Management Study – Indian Institute of Management Ahmedabad:

In a move to propel the institution's future growth, the Council commissioned a comprehensive study by the Indian Institute of Management, Ahmedabad (IIM–A) in October 1988. This initiative aimed to develop a roadmap for CMC Vellore's trajectory in the years ahead. The IIM–A team undertook an evaluation of the institution's financial policies and overall fiscal health. Significantly, the study concluded that the expansion into various specialised medical services, as envisioned by the faculty, was not only sound but also financially viable. This endorsement from a prestigious management institute provided a critical foundation for CMC Vellore's planned diversification into specific medical specialties. However, the success of such an undertaking hinged not only on financial feasibility but also on the unwavering commitment of both staff and administration. The long-term vision and dedication of all stakeholders would be paramount to ensuring the sustainability of these ambitious endeavours.

3. Continuing Medical Education (CME):

Recognising the critical importance of continuous professional development, Dr. Pulimood began the Continuing Medical Education (CME) programme near the end of his tenure as Director. The CME programme aimed to equip doctors with the latest medical knowledge and skills. By providing ongoing educational opportunities, the programme ensured that CMC Vellore's physicians remained abreast of contemporary advancements in their respective fields. This, in turn, empowered them to deliver the highest quality of care to their patients. Dr. Pulimood's foresight in implementing this vital programme ensured that CMC Vellore would continue to be a leader in providing exceptional medical education.

Stalwarts Retire

Amidst the bustling currents of change, Dr. LBM Joseph, a stalwart in the medical realm, gracefully stepped into the twilight of his career.His tenure had been etched with the ink of dedication and merit. Yes, it was during a tempestuous chapter that Dr. Joseph's leadership came to the forefront. A prolonged and relentless strike by a faction of the staff threatened to cast shadows upon the Institution's harmony.

Sensitive and strong leadership of Dr. Joseph had brought in a new atmosphere of tranquillity and peace in the institution.

The retirement of Dr. KV Mathai made one reflect on past events. It is crucial to acknowledge Dr. Mathai's contributions and the unforeseen chain of events triggered by his arrest during the strike. Holding the esteemed position of neurosurgeon to the then Prime Minister, Mrs. Indira Gandhi, Dr. Mathai's situation garnered national attention. Recognising the potential impact on CMC Vellore, Prime Minister Mrs. Gandhi dispatched Mr. Sanjeev Reddy to Madras (now Chennai) with a clear mandate to resolve the ongoing strike. Mr. Reddy's swift intervention involved direct communication with the Chief Minister, Mr. Karunanidhi. The following day, a momentous decision unfolded. The strike, which had paralysed normalcy, was ordered to be withdrawn. And where did this resolution take place? Within the very halls of the State Legislative Assembly! The crippling strike was officially called off.

Dr. Pulimood's term as Director was from 1987–1993. Dr. Pulimood's leadership qualities were evident even during his youth. As captain of the Kerala State Football Team, he displayed a remarkable aptitude for leadership. While a position like forward might garner more glory through scoring goals, Dr. Pulimood chose the role of goalkeeper – the team's last line of defense. This deliberate selection epitomised his unwavering commitment to protecting and supporting his team, even in the face of adversity. This selfless characteristic foreshadowed his leadership style as Director of the Christian Medical College and Hospital. Much like a skilled goalkeeper, Dr. Pulimood excelled at safeguarding the Institution's well-being. His dedication to both medical education and patient care remained steadfast throughout his tenure. Under his visionary guidance, CMC Vellore achieved significant progress, solidifying its position as a premier healthcare and educational institution.

Chapter 12

An Instrument of God's Love and Care for His Sick and Needy Children

Dr. V I Mathan

At the end of Benjamin Pulimood's term as Director, the search committee for his successor identified me as possessing the necessary skills and experience, however there was a potential problem as I had only 3 ½ years till I retired at the age of 60. The committee considered giving me a full seven–year term as Director to ensure maximum contribution to the Institution. I was absolutely clear that under no circumstances was I going to violate the rules and traditions of the Institution by staying on beyond the age of sixty. The committee, without further discussion, accepted my stand and appointed me as the Director till my time of superannuation. My term was from March 1994 to September 1997.

In the next 3 ½ years, I tried to achieve all that I envisioned for the development of the Institution. When I spelt out my plan to the Executive Committee, they were sceptical that even half of it could be achieved in the 3 ½ years. I wanted to:

1. Streamline and make the administration of the institution more efficient.

2. Facilitate the various departments and units to attain their full potential by fostering an atmosphere of excellence within the Institution.

3. Encourage individual development and recruit new faculty in identified areas of need.

4. Plan and develop new departments as appropriate.

5. Strengthen the alumni network.

The next 3 ½ years were in some ways, the busiest years of my life. Six days a week, I would leave home around 7 AM in the morning and return after 8 PM. Even on Sundays, after the morning service at Fort Church, I would be in the office to catch up on the week's correspondence, leaving tapes with dictated letters for the secretaries to type in the morning.

The words of my mentor, Mr. Thomas Abraham, that the captain of the team does not play alone, were constantly in my mind. Dr. Samraj who was then an Assistant Director was, at my request, appointed as the Associate Director. He very efficiently dealt with the routine responsibilities of the office in consultation with me. This gave me sufficient time to interact with all the staff who wanted to share their concerns with me and make suggestions for improving the Institution.

Since I had visited every unit and department in the Institution as the Medical Superintendent, I had a good understanding of the spectrum of concern and could respond to them appropriately. It was my policy that the Director's office door was always open for any staff member to walk in and present their problem. I would then suggest a solution and dictate an appropriate letter into the dictaphone. On an average day, the secretaries had 20 to 40 such letters to type.

The actual administration of each area of the Institution was left to the individual administrative officers, who had access to me any time if they so desired, either by phone or in person. I must thank and congratulate my colleagues who discharged these responsibilities efficiently and faithfully.

The Administrative Committee meetings, every Thursday, were an excellent opportunity to review these issues. At 6 PM, if the meeting was not concluded, the AC would decide who was responsible for the delay and that person had to pay for the second round of coffee and snacks. Unfortunately, the usual culprit was myself!

Administrative changes

One of the biggest concerns was to bring our administration on par with the best that is needed for an institution of our size. A policy that administrative officers who are involved in formulating policy (the director, principal, and the medical superintendent) should be health professionals is crucial to the success of the institution. Since these are full–time or almost full–time posts, it is a difficult decision for skilled healthcare professionals to give up their clinical work and take up administration. A question has been asked many times and will be asked many more times – Should we not handover the administration to professional administrators? This experiment has been tried in the other large healthcare organisations and found to be ineffective. However, at the same time, we needed to have a large number of professional administrators to carry out our policies. One of the problems was that we could not attract many such professionals, although we thank God for the few who have joined the Institution with commitment. It is our policy now to encourage the development of middle level managers in the hope that some or many of them would come up to senior administrative positions in due course of time. A good career structure was provided for such individuals.

An important matter to remember in administration is that we have to be a truly democratic institution. True democracy means that knowledge has to be in the hands of all the people so that lack of knowledge does not lead to a dictatorial style of functioning. An administrative handbook was developed during my period, which would make necessary information available to all faculty and staff.

I made crucial changes to further strengthen the administration. Dr. Chakko Korula Jacob, who previously held the Deputy Director position, assumed additional responsibilities by taking the reins of the Medical Superintendent's Office. Furthermore, I recognised the potential of Dr. Jasper Daniel, a medical microbiologist, then on sabbatical leave in England. I actively encouraged him to return from his leave early so that he would be available in Vellore when the then General Superintendent retired. This proved to be a successful move, as Dr. Daniel, upon his return, served as the General Superintendent with great distinction until his retirement. The General Superintendent had a massive responsibility when taken into consideration, the 8,000 employees, over 1,000 doctors, about 1,000 technical people, around 2,000 office staff and another 2,200 class 3 and class 4 employees and all the staff of the college campus, besides college staff, secretarial staff, attenders and technicians. The General Superintendent was responsible to see that these people worked properly, that they were efficient and at the same time happy to work.

The term of Dr. Bhooshanam as Principal was completed, and Dr. Joyce Ponnaiya was appointed to this critical position.

Realising that it would be necessary to have at least a crore of rupees from Vellore as the core of the century fund, Dr. AS Kanagasabapathy, Professor of Biochemistry, was appointed by me for this purpose. Dr. Kanagasabapathy had an exceptional talent for public relation, a skill set crucial for a successful fundraising campaign. He spearheaded this effort, getting a remarkable initial contribution of over a crore of rupees from the town of Vellore. He was an effective and persuasive advocate for the Institution.

I have been privileged to work with three treasurers of our Institution, Mr. CC Jacob, Mr. G Jesudian and Mr. Manickam. God has blessed us by giving us people with high integrity, total commitment to Christ and an equally total commitment towards the Institution to be at the helm of our financial affairs.

An affirmation of education

A critical element in Aunt Ida's vision was the central role of education and teaching as the core of our institution. We have a large number of training programmes in three faculties, medical, nursing and allied health services. It was a major consideration whether we should try and be a "deemed to be" university. However, it was not clear whether "deemed to be" university could also be a minority educational institution. After careful consideration, we decided to continue to be affiliated to the State University. While this restricts our ability to be innovative in education, it protects the real benefits of being a minority educational institution. This allows us to admit Christian students predominantly and have a faculty that is mainly Christian and an administration that is wholly Christian.

Faculty development and research

Several new clinical and service departments were started to improve our patient care services. This included Neonatology, Clinical Virology, Endocrinology, Reproductive Medicine, and Developmental Paediatrics. Existing staff were further trained or new faculty were recruited for starting these clinical initiatives.

Dr. MC Matthew, a renowned specialist from Chennai with extensive experience working with children with developmental problems was persuaded by me to relocate to Vellore, which he did. This strategic move marked a significant milestone for CMCH, as it represented the first instance of a fully developed specialty being brought in from outside. Unlike other institutions that developed specialties internally over time, CMCH acquired a department that was already established and operational. This forward–thinking decision positioned Developmental Paediatrics as one of CMCH's strongest departments.

To ensure that our teaching and services are at the cutting edge, all faculty are encouraged to take an opportunity to enhance the skill in other centres up to three years. This study leave also enables them to improve their financial resources. In addition, every five years faculty members can accumulate sabbatical leave, which can be accumulated over a period of 15 years to a maximum three years. A new facility, which was introduced by me, was for the senior professors to get special deputation up to six months with full pay, either to learn a new skill or enhance their professional skills.

All along, I had been concerned looking at earlier senior administrators that their seven years term of service was too long, and that after five years, their efforts slackened and several appeared to be coasting. After a long discussion with all the administrative staff and professional staff, we decided that the term of a senior administrator recruited from the faculty should be for a maximum of five years and not renewed. The concept of the rotating headship of units of departments was discussed individually with every professional staff by me and was presented to the Council and accepted by them. This is now being implemented.

Research

The research at Vellore was focussed on problems relevant to our country. We had a few groups whose work received national and international recognition. Individual faculty members made significant contributions to solving relevant public health problems. It was interesting that the milieu of Vellore encouraged a non–clinical faculty, Dr. James Verghese, who started the Department of Chemistry for the few years we had a pre–medical course to continue on after that, and established himself as a major researcher with ten doctoral graduates.

Innovative, compassionate technology

The honourable Shri KR Narayanan, when he was inaugurating our first magnetic resonance image scanner in 1995, coined the term "compassionate technology" to describe what he and his wife had experienced in Vellore Hospital. The vision of Aunt Ida *that the Institution should be self-supporting makes the use of high technology essential to ensure revenue generation. The unique attribute at Vellore is the use of technology to express Christ's compassion and love for patients. The example of this is an innovative approach to perform mitral valvotomy through a trans-septal approach using a balloon* catheter, which reduced the hospital stay, expenses and inconvenience to the patients for this common clinical condition.

A continuing commitment to the poor

While it is essential to the Institution to have high paying patients to maintain the finances, there is a continuing commitment that about 1/5th of our operating budget is for the care of poor patients. We also provide enough scholarships to ensure that 1/3rd of the students in the degree programme (medical and nursing) and almost half the students in other education programmes are from economically disadvantaged sections of the society. Generous scholarships are provided for such students. In addition to this, the cost of free and subsidised care is equivalent to the budget of a government district hospital, mainly provided to poor patients from our immediate vicinity.

The financial self-sufficiency of our Institution, which enables us to do large amounts of charitable work as well as subsidise our educational endeavours to the tune of almost fifty lakhs is the result of the vision of Aunt Ida that provision of care of the highest order, especially specialised care would generate income from our country, which can then be used for treating the needy, the marginalised and the poor as well as for educating more students in the ideals of our Institution. She initiated this process by starting the Department of Neurosurgery and

Thoracic Surgery. If we divide the decade since 1987 into the first five years and the next five years, we invested 13.7% of the maintenance expenditure in equipment during the first five years which increased to 19.7% in the last five years. This trend has to be maintained to ensure the viability of the infrastructure. Most institutions' approach to finance management is to keep aside a significant reserve. If we now invest money, with constraints on us, the maximum return is likely to be at the most 15%. However, a perusal of the expenditure and income statement clearly shows that the increased investment in the Institution has resulted in significant financial returns. During the last three years, we have re-organised the way in which interest-bearing and interest-free internal loans are used with very clear guidelines that have been approved by the Executive Committee and are closely monitored at three-monthly intervals. There is sufficient flexibility to ensure that the growth and development of our Institution will not be hampered. We have also used external loans judiciously when necessary, a policy which was initiated at the time by my predecessor, BM Pulimood.

A very important policy of our Institution that must be emphasised is that all external grants and donations are totally used for the stated purpose and no form of administrative charge is levied. This I understand is unique among charitable organisations and is a true measure of our financial stewardship.

24/7 hospital

As development and growth were happening, there were other significant things taking place. The staff were given a free hand to take many initiatives. If a staff had new ideas for an initiative, they were encouraged. They felt empowered by the sense of full freedom to do whatever they wanted and many stepped forward with ideas. In many institutions, leaders often feel threatened when others take on new initiatives. However, here an ecosystem was created to foster and encourage original ideas.

The routine activities of the Institution had to go on. As things improved, word got around to patients that if you go to Vellore, you will get very good treatment. So, patient numbers more than doubled in those three and a half years. In fact, the total number became three times more. New staff had to be recruited into the Hospital. Fortunately, there was no problem on this front. Although there was a struggle to accommodate all the patients, the Institute managed to provide good quality service for all.

The next step in enhancing patient care involved streamlining the appointment process to prioritise patient convenience. This pioneering effort by CMCH manifested in the introduction of 24–hour appointment scheduling for essential services. While the concept of a 24–hour hospital is commonplace today, it is crucial to recognise the revolutionary nature of this approach in 1995, particularly within the context of Vellore. At that time, such extended access to healthcare services was a novel idea and a significant advancement for patient accessibility.

CMCH's Alumni Network: A Cornerstone of Growth

Over the years, CMCH had cultivated an exceptionally strong alumni network that became a cornerstone of its continued growth and success. This network flourished to the point where nearly 95% of the faculty were former CMCH students. This remarkable statistic placed CMCH in a league of its own, boasting one of the highest percentages of alumni contribution among academic institutions. They have contributed to the vibrancy of our witness and ministry by their work wherever they are in the world.

This robust alumni network offered a multitude of benefits. It ensured a steady influx of talented faculty members who possessed a deep understanding of CMCH's values and mission. These individuals were inherently invested in the Institution's success, having themselves benefited from its world–class education. The administration's role, therefore, became one of identifying promising students who demonstrated a strong potential to contribute meaningfully to CMCH's legacy. Once identified, persuading these individuals to remain at Vellore became a key objective.

While the limitations of Vellore as a city, with its relatively fewer entertainment options compared to metropolitan areas, presented a challenge, a sense of commitment ultimately prevailed. The dedication of faculty stemmed from a deep desire to contribute to CMCH's mission and propel it to even greater heights. This commitment transcended external factors, solidifying the alumni network's position as a vital force in CMCH's enduring success.

One of my concerns when I took the responsibility of the Director was to get to know the staff better and get them to interact with each other in a non–professional setting. The Chairman of the Council was also the Chair of the Ecumenical Christian Council Centre in Whitefield, outside Bangalore, and made their facilities available to us. We were able to identify

Rev. Valsan Thampu, who was in Saint Stephens College, Delhi, as an inspirational speaker, who conducted weekend retreats for groups of around 30 to 35 staff members almost every month. We would leave Vellore on Friday afternoon and return on Sunday afternoon. I attended all the retreats and the feedback was very valuable in planning the progress of the Institution. Nearly 35 such retreats covered almost all the faculty. This was an opportunity for free exchange of ideas away from Vellore and allowed people from different areas of the Institution to get to know each other better.

One day, as I was signing the papers for paying the pension of an attendant, who was retiring after 40 years of service, something struck my mind that this person was getting a pension of Rs. 4000/– per month, which was actually the salary of senior professors at the time of retirement in the 1960s. In consultation with the Treasurer, I devised a new plan for the pension scheme which is now in operation. This ensures that with each salary revision, the pension is also adjusted guaranteeing that it never falls below the entitled proportion based on the new pay scale.

I was very conscious of the fact that the year 2000 would be the centenary year of Aunt Ida starting work at Vellore in 1900 January. Although I was to retire three years prior to that, it was essential that planning and preparation started well in advance to.celebrate the centenary appropriately. I therefore involved all my colleagues in administration as well as senior faculty in actively planning, and preparing for this event.

I had left a detailed document outlining my dreams about the centenary celebration and the preparation I had started. This included major construction including accommodation for staff and house surgeons, staff nurses' hostel and a centre for women and children. It was envisaged that Alumni, particularly those overseas, should be a major source of funds. It is gratifying that the US alumni, committed more than half of what we had hoped to collect.

I specially mention, Dr. Pulimood, Dr. Samraj, Dr. Punnoose Matthew, Mr. Manickam, Mr. Jesudian, Dr. Kanagasabapathy, Dr. Joyce Ponnaiya, Dr. Matthew Chandy, Dr. Jasper Daniel, Mr. JK Madhuranayagam and Dr. Prasanna Rajan as people who require special thanks. To my friends, Prakash Khanduri and Shankar Krishna Swamy, who helped me more than they know, thank you. The Council and particularly the members of the Executive Committee and Finance Committee have been my source of strength. The brotherly affection and concern, particularly of Dr. Mithra Augustine, Bishop Elia Peter, Dr. MA Thangarajh, Dr. Esho John, Mr. Thomas Abraham, Dr. JC Vijayan, Dr. Ajith Singh, Rev. Valsan Thambu and Dr. J Krishmukti among many others is what sustained me; I will not say thank you as I know you are as much a part of the Institution as I am. From among my teachers, I would specially like to thank Professor P Kutumbiah, Principal when I joined this Institution for inspiring me to be a physician, Padma Bhushan Professor Jacob Chandy and Professor JC David, who convinced me the necessity of efficient administration and Professor Selwyn Baker, who guided me in my first steps in research and Professor KI Vithilingam who was my inspiration in becoming a good clinician.

The Christian Medical College and Hospital Vellore is an expression of the Church's commitment to Christ's Healing Ministry. We serve all in need of healing without consideration of caste and creed with a special commitment to the poor, the needy and the marginalised. We accept financial viability from God through the effective utilisation of our skills, training young men, and women in the spirit of Christ, using technology as a gift from God to further His Healing Ministry. We express the highest standards of integrity, fellowship, compassion and skill so that the fruits of the spirit, love, joy, peace, patience, kindness, goodness, faithfulness, humility, and self–control will be a beacon to our nation.

As we went forward toward the new millennium, I was confident that God would give us the wisdom to realise the true dimension of our role and help us to develop strategies and plans which will move us towards this goal.

I handed over the responsibilities of the Director's Office to Prof. Joyce Ponnaiya, who had started her career as a research fellow in my Unit. She was the Principal of the College during the latter half of my term and was well aware of the plans and programmes for the Centenary and was an active participant in the preparation. I happily handed over all responsibilities to her on the evening before my 60th birthday, after a public function led by Bishop Elia Peter, thanking God for my services and installing Joyce as the next Director. I signed the last few papers and spent the next three months completing all the work in the Wellcome Unit, while waiting for my wife to retire. We left for Bangladesh at the end of December 1997 and I joined as the Associate Director of Laboratory Services at the International Centre for Diarrhoeal Disease Research, Dhaka. We spent the next three years there and then went to Delhi to spend a year at UNAIDS. We returned and settled in Chennai.

Appendix 1

The Pioneers Who Prepared the Ground

Why did a successful young New York Physician, Dr. John Scudder, suddenly renounce the good life he enjoyed and leave for India on a sailing ship, the Indus, in June 1819 with his wife and two–year–old daughter? He was the first American Medical Missionary to India.

Tracing Dr. John's parentage helps to understand his motivation. His paternal grandfather, Dr. Nathaniel Scudder, was an American patriot who was a member of the Continental Congress which declared independence from England. When the war started, he was commissioned Colonel in the Monmouth Militia and served as a battle front doctor throughout the War of Independence. Three days before the surrender of English forces, he got news that a skirmish was taking place nearby and he volunteered to go and bind up the wounded. While he was attending to the wounded, a stray bullet killed him, the only member of the Continental Congress to die in the War of Independence. His maternal grandfather, Colonel Philip Johnston, when ordered to storm an impregnable British position, first pointed out the futility of the attempt and then led his men to a battle doomed to failure with only one of them surviving! This was Dr. John's heritage of duty and discipline.

Maria Johnston Scudder, Dr. John's mother, instilled the essence of Christianity in her children and taught them that life was not indulgence but disciplined attention to duty. Joseph Scudder, the father, was a distinguished and successful lawyer. John wanted to be ordained for the ministry but his father forbade him to follow that path and was happy that he chose to become a doctor in his grandfather's footsteps. John Scudder, the second of twelve children to his parents, was born on September 3rd 1793, graduated from Princeton in 1811 and received his medical degree from the College of Physicians of New York in 1815. During his college days, his nickname was 'Goodman Scudder' because of his serious Christian behaviour and his striving to be what his mother instilled in him. He began his practice in New York City and by 1819 had gained quite a reputation by his ability to gain the confidence of his patients, clinical skills and kindness.

Dr. John started his New York practice staying as a boarder in the home of Mrs. Gideon Waterbury. He was concerned that they were not devout enough as Christians and he reasoned with them to bring them to a greater commitment. His success led to his marrying the eldest daughter, Harriet Waterbury who was lovely in person, gentle, joyous and practical. She was indeed a leaven in the life of the all too serious John. Their daughter, Maria was two years old in 1819 when John was challenged by reading a tract on the necessity of taking the Christian Gospel to far lands, in the parlour of one of his patients. John, whose first choice of career had been to be ordained as a minister, felt compelled to offer himself as a medical missionary. But first he had to get the concurrence of Harriet. It was not an easy decision, but finally her love for her husband, her own Christian commitment and sense of duty won and she agreed to go with him to an unknown land. His father disinherited him for daring to be a missionary. Dr. John offered himself as a medical missionary to the American Board of Commissioners for Foreign Missions and accepted their appointment on 1 May 1819, five weeks before he, Harriet, Maria and a devoted black maid Amy, along with three other missionary families sailed into the unknown, trusting the Lord who had called them.

The four–month journey from Boston to Calcutta was uneventful but tedious. Dr. John took upon himself the task of bringing the sailors on the ship to give a commitment to be devout Christians. All accepted his exhortations prior to their landing in Calcutta but regrettably most reverted back to their old habits soon after the temptations of the port were available!

Calcutta to Jaffna

It must have been with great relief that the four missionary families moved into a house in Calcutta for a two–month stay before proceeding to their final destination, Jaffna in northern Ceylon (now Sri Lanka). This interlude, necessitated by the birth of a baby to one of the families onboard the ship, was welcomed by the missionaries as it gave them a chance to visit Dr. William Carey, pioneer missionary and theologian at Serampore near Calcutta. Dr. John and his colleagues learnt much about the nuts and bolts of running a mission from this pioneer.

Unfortunately in Calcutta, Maria their infant daughter was struck by dysentery and died within three days, an event that devastated the young parents but did not change their commitment or resolve. In a letter to his mother immediately after the tragedy, he wrote:

"O My Dear Mother, how shall I take up my pen to mark upon paper the dark shadow of death? My dear little babe is no more. She has left us for ever... This is a heartrending trial; but we can say and do say 'The will of the Lord be done'. My dear Harriet bears it remarkably well. Oh my Mother, had she, the dearest object of my affection been called away how dark and desolate I would have been! Pray for us; we need Divine support more than you are aware."

This poignant letter documenting their great loss, shows their deep commitment to the call they had embarked on, the strength that Dr. John drew from his wife Harriet and his deep love for her and their absolute dependence on the Lord through prayer.

The two months in Calcutta soon passed, and the group embarked for Colombo for onward travel to Jaffna. En route, as the ship was passing the port of Trincomalee on the east coast of Ceylon, Dr. John was requested to disembark and go by a land route to Jaffna where one of the American missionaries was in urgent need of his help. The 150 miles to Jaffna was covered in about a week on foot, porters carrying their luggage and Harriet and Dr. John carried in palanquins borne on the shoulders of porters. They journeyed by night as the days were too hot. Their way was lit by flaming torches, and the porters sang along to break the tedium of the way and to keep the wild animals away. When they reached Jaffna, they were welcomed by the missionaries and found that the patient had terminal tuberculosis for which nothing could be done, a common problem among the missionaries.

Teaching and Healing in Jaffna, Panditeripo and Chavagacherry 1820 – 1836

The American Mission to Jaffna had started four schools in Jaffna in the four years they had been working there. Dr. John was the first American or any other medical person to practice in Ceylon (now Sri Lanka). The strength of their commitment to the mission is seen from a letter home soon after the death of their second daughter a week after her birth:

"After breathing the tainted air for but one week, she closed her eyes upon us forever, and took her flight to join her beloved sister. This is a severe trial, but we do not repine. We, however, must have the feelings of nature. We must say our trials have been heart–rending. Perhaps, our dear parents may be ready (for us) to say that we are sorry and repent of our coming. No, we rejoice and thank the Great Head of the Church for putting into our hearts to leave America and come and live among this people. I would not exchange situations for a world.

Blessed be the Lord, I hope to be the unworthy instrument of bringing souls to the Redeemer."

Their third child, a son, also died soon after birth in 1821, and still, there was no sense of regret on their chosen path. Mrs. Harriet was her husband's full partner and committed to the alleviation of the misery of the poorest of the poor in the land to which they had been sent by their Redeemer.

Apart from the infections that killed off their first three children, they had to learn how to bring their children up in the tropical heat, humidity, dirt, termites, snakes, scorpions, ants, spiders and many other perils with very limited facilities and money. The rapidity of their learning curve is shown by the fact that the fourth child, Henry Martin, born to them in Panditeripo in 1822, and the fifth, William Waterbury, born in 1823, both survived and thrived. A further eight children – six boys and two girls – were born, the youngest boy, John Scudder II, in October 1836 and Louisa, the second surviving daughter, a year later. It would be easy to assume that with ten children born in a period of fifteen years, Mrs Harriet would have no time for doing anything other than look after them and bring them up in a hostile environment. The record speaks otherwise.

Dr. John was driven by his passionate commitment to winning souls for Christ. Medicine was a means to an end, an entry point to preach the Gospel to those who came to him for help. He believed that he would be held accountable for every soul he met whom he didn't strive to bring to the full knowledge and acceptance of Christ. His day started at sunrise, and he spent an hour and a half in prayer and Bible study. The patients would collect from the town and surrounding areas, first listen to his biblical exhortation, and then be treated. He had learnt sufficient Tamil to read scholarly works and preach to his patients as well as in marketplaces. We do not have a record of how many souls he won but his passion for his calling is shown by the long hours he preached under the burning sun in market places, the many insults he endured without any reaction and his stringency in evaluating those who claimed they were believers before baptising them. Perhaps, he was influenced by the memory of what happened to the sailors on Indus who claimed they were a new creation, soon after their arrival in Calcutta. He was ordained a Pastor in 1821 in a Wesleyan chapel in Jaffna by the locally available congregational, baptist and methodist ministers, probably the first ecumenical activity of the Church in India.

Equal importance was given to starting schools where a Christian education was given. Since the Board did not provide adequate funds, the Scudders used their own sparse resources to start the work without thought of where more money would come for the family. Dr. John and Mrs. Harriet started with two schools in Panditeripo, one for boys and another for girls. It was difficult to persuade families to send their girls to school. Boys from nearby areas attended mainly as day scholars but attendees from further away and all girls boarded with the Scudders. Any orphaned children they found were also offered school and boarding. There were times when as many as 45 children, in addition to her own, were looked after by Mrs. Harriet. She was ably assisted in this by the maid Amy. It is a pity that we do not know much about her and her work and in fact what happened to her. Once, Amy became very sick and they considered sending her back to America but she recovered and continued her devoted service. She was still there when William, the second son, came back to work as a missionary in Jaffna in the early 1840s. Where did they find teachers for these schools? One of the schools in Jaffna was ultimately elevated to the status of a degree giving college and a seminary to train teachers and evangelists. Dr. John trained several boys to assist him in the care of patients as his assistants, a tradition followed by his sons.

This small beginning out of necessity came to full flower when his granddaughter started the Missionary Medical School for Women at Vellore almost a hundred years later.

What was the nature of his work as a Doctor? Looking back, we have to remember that Dr. John was one of the earliest practitioners of 'modern medicine' in India in the pre–antibiotic, pre-anaesthetic and pre-evidence based medicine era nearly 200 years ago. He excised tumours and there is an anecdote of a twelve-year-old girl from whose back he excised two tumours through an eight-inch long incision, who continued to shout choicest epithets at him during the process. Pulling out infected or broken teeth, setting broken bones, amputations, repairing torn ear lobes and removing cataracts were other surgical treatments. The cataract surgery was most successful, but to his dismay many patients came to him after they had the opaque lens pushed back into the vitreous by indigenous practitioners resulting in inflammation and permanent blindness. A variety of fevers which must have included malaria, typhoid and tuberculosis and epidemics of cholera, confronted him. Specific therapies, which are now widely available were unknown then and the patients were managed by tender loving care and supportive measures. His prescription for cholera was five grains of powdered opium and fifteen grains of calomel followed by a cathartic a few hours later, provided the patient survived that long! Dr. John and when they returned home for lunch, their cook had just returned after burying his wife who died of cholera and after he served them lunch he died in their kitchen. Dr. John's reaction was to fumigate their kitchen which was interpreted many as offering incense to propitiate their God! All infectious disease was believed to be the punishment of particular gods or goddesses and all that could be done was to try and propitiate them. There are records in indigenous medicine of treating cholera by giving a ball of opium to the patient and when it was vomited out wash it and force the patient to swallow it again repeatedly till either the patient died or the opium stayed down which was the harbinger of recovery, a very rare event!

Dr. John did not confine his medical and evangelistic efforts to Panditeripo and Jaffna. Once it was well established there, he extended it to surrounding villages, nearby districts and outlying islands. Dr. John was away from Panditeripo for days or weeks at a time as he would take his medicines, Bible and tracts (apparently inscribed on dried palm leaves) and travel to other villages and to the nearby islands. Travel was not a pleasurable exercise. Carried on bullock carts or palanquins through surrounding jungles, wading across streams and rivers, going to nearby islands by small rowing boats some with a single sail and staying the nights usually under the shade of his umbrella to keep the dew away from his head, it was his passion for propagating the gospel that drove Dr. John. Away from the limited comforts of his home, he started to fall ill with severe headaches and bouts of fever, probably malaria which were diagnosed as jungle fever. Standing for long periods under the sun to preach the gospel at public markets did not help to improve his health. At many such events, he was heckled and waste was thrown at him. He patiently endured all this as essential to his mission, but it did not improve his health. The interludes at Panditeripo in a thatched hut with mud floors did little to recharge him. His zeal for his mission drove him much beyond his strength. The steady deterioration of his health was a matter of concern and by 1829, his health had deteriorated to such an extent that the mission sent Dr. John and family to recuperate in the cool climate of the Nilgiris in mainland India. The family stayed there for over a year and returned to Panditeripo by September 1830.

Their financial limitation meant that food was mainly rice and vegetables they had grown in the kitchen garden Mrs. Harriet cultivated. She also developed a flower garden and all this was watered from the 20–foot deep well they had dug.

An interesting footnote is that ropes were placed around the thatched mud floored 'bungalow' they lived in to keep out the snakes who apparently did not like to crawl over the rough coir ropes! Mrs. Harriet would be left alone to supervise the schools, visit patients treated by Dr. John to follow up, look after her own children and the boarders and ensure that the work at the mission continued without interruption during the periods Dr. John was away taking the gospel to surrounding areas. There is no record of any complaint by Mrs. Harriet of the difficulties that she faced. She was the true heroine of the Scudder Mission to India, uncomplainingly shouldering all that was to be done to make their mission succeed. The accomplishment of her life is the service to India by her ten surviving children and the success of Dr. John's mission.

The Scudder Ministry continued at Panditeripo. It was clear that there was no future for their children if they continued to grow up in India and the Board was persuaded to provide for sending them back to United States of America where hopefully they would be looked after and educated by their relatives. The values instilled in them by Dr. John and Mrs. Harriet ensured that all the boys completed college, were ordained, and four of them were medically qualified. Unfortunately one of them, Samuel born in 1827, died in a drowning accident while training at a seminary preparing to come back to India. The seven surviving sons and the two daughters returned to work as missionaries in India. The eldest Henry Martyn, seminary educated, soon after his return to India realised the value of medical work and was qualified from the newly started Madras Medical College.

Dr. John and Mrs. Harriet handed over the well-established mission station at Panditeripo to a newly arrived doctor in 1834 and moved to Chavagacherry to start a new mission station. Here, they had to start anew and replicate and build on what they had done at Panditeripo and the Scudders uncomplainingly took up the task. The Jaffna Mission received further workers and so the Board decided in 1836 that Dr. John, Mrs. Harriet and family should relocate to Madras, the then seat of British Rule in southern India.

Madras and a visit Home, 1836 to 1846

How much the decision to shift Dr. John and family to Madras was influenced by his health is not clear. Recurrent attacks of Jungle fever, repeated bouts of diarrhoea and persistent chronic headache had undermined his health. His commitment to his work was such that he drove himself in the quest of souls. Ceylon in those days was just a province of India and the decision for the transfer was probably influenced by the thought that in metropolitan Madras with a large expatriate population and possible cultural opportunities, the pace at which he was driving himself would be slower and his health may recover to an extent. At Madras, his target was to establish a Christian higher educational institution in partnership with other missionaries. He formed a partnership with Dr. Anderson of the Church of Scotland for this and travelled extensively to try and raise funds. Wherever he went, he would also preach and use his medical skills as an entry point for the Gospel. Travelling by bullock cart or palanquin with just a few young men he had trained and paucity of accommodation were all telling on his health. By 1841, his health was so bad that he was sent to the Nilgiris for recuperation but this did not help him and it was decided in March 1842, twenty–three years after they had sailed from Boston, the Scudders, Dr. John, Mrs. Harriet and five younger children were on a ship going back home around the Cape of Good Hope. The five older boys were already in school there.

The long ship journey partially restored Dr. John's health. The high point of his return was the reconciliation with his father. The four years they spent in America were used by Dr. John to travel extensively and to talk to Church groups and schools on the great need for missionary work. He was a good speaker and particularly effective with children. However, while his health improved, he had a persistent cough. Four years later in November 1846, Dr. John, Mrs. Harriet and his second son, William and his bride and the two daughters sailed for India. They reached Madras in March to be greeted by their first son Henry Martyn and his wife and the news of the death of their newborn son.

Madras, Madurai, Pudukottai and Vellore

An outbreak of cholera in Madurai saw Dr. John being sent there to tackle it, but nothing had changed in the management of cholera and it continued to be the great killer. Dr. John continued to travel and had a particularly delightful interlude with the Raja of Pudukottai, where he stayed for several months and did many successful surgeries and developed a very good relationship with the Raja, whom he tried to convince to be a Christian. Dr. John became embroiled in the caste controversy as part of the life of the Church while in Madurai and took a strong stance against caste being recognised by the Church. This controversy continued and his sons were equally convinced that recognising caste among Christians was against the essence of the Gospel. This controversy still continues. Dr. John in his extensive travels visited Vellore, which he recognised as an excellent field for

Christian work. His prophetic description of Vellore was fulfilled when his granddaughter started her work there in 1900.

Dr. John and family returned to Madras in 1849 and were greeted by the death of Kate, wife of their second son William, and soon thereafter by news of the death of their fourth son Samuel in a drowning accident while in a seminary in the USA. A greater tragedy was to follow. Mrs. Harriet, who had heroically borne the burden of their life in the tropics, suddenly became ill. It is not clear what she suffered from as all that is known is that she had cramps, severe exhaustion and unbearable sensitivity if anybody touched her. She was ill for four days and died on November 18, 1949. The loss of his beloved wife, companion, and staunch supporter was a blow from which Dr. John did not recover. He continued to work harder than ever, preaching the Gospel three times a day and attending to patients with his son Henry. His health steadily deteriorated and the Mission decided to send him to Capetown in 1854 to recover, as he refused to be repatriated to the USA. He continued to preach there and the local dailies reported the amazing response from children of all races to his message. On 13 January 1855, he preached in the morning and quietly went to his Master while resting before he was to preach again in the evening. His body was brought back to Madras and buried next to his wife.

In Memorium

Sixty–two years, thirty in the USA and thirty–two in India, what is the legacy of this life that CMC Vellore should celebrate?

A committed disciplined life fuelled by the burning desire to win souls to Christ, spending himself in pursuit of his goal without counting the cost, practising the state–of–the–art in medical care and the ability to inspire others to the same commitment are the hallmarks of Dr. John's life. His legacy was established by his children coming back to serve in India, inspite of the hardships they grew up in. Dr. John and Mrs. Harriet and their children and grandchildren gave over a thousand years in–service in India. Dr. John's life was crowned by his granddaughter Ida Sophia establishing the Christian Medical College in Vellore, which has amplified the thousand years of service to India by the Scudder family manyfold. The continuing generations at Vellore should commit themselves anew to follow the Master's charge to "Heal and Teach". There is much in the life of Dr. John and Mrs. Harriet for the succeeding generations to celebrate.

Fertilised and Watered

The unique inheritance that Dr. John and Mrs. Harriet left was their nine surviving children who came back to work in India. The words of Henry, the eldest, describe their affair with India:

> *"India's bright skies, sunny plains and luxuriant foliage have a charm for me… I love India, I love her soil, I love her people."*

This was true for all the children. The two daughters returned as missionaries but they soon married Englishmen and moved away from the Mission. The seven surviving sons were ordained ministers and five of them medically trained. They were responsible for starting the Arcot Mission which was the base for Aunt Ida's work from the beginning of the twentieth century.

Henry Martyn Scudder

Henry was sent back to the States when he was ten years old and was under the care of Jared Waterbury, his mother's brother. He wanted to enrol in Princeton like all his family but finances decided that he join New York University. At the end of the first year, he was withdrawn from the University and enrolle himself at Williamstown from where he was also withdrawn and sent to his grandparents where he worked as a farm labourer. His uncle, Rev. Downer however met him and discovered great hidden potential in him. Rev. Downer persuaded New York University to admit him with a scholarship. This act of love transformed him and he graduated, married Fanny Lewis and left in 1844 as a missionary to India. Soon after his arrival in Madras, he realised the value of medical training in his work and took instruction from the newly started Madras Medical College and was able to work with his father when he returned to India in 1847. Four years later, he moved with his family to Wallajah where he initially ran a clinic and did surgery but his real interest was in preaching the Gospel. Three years later, when a government dispensary was opened nearby, he spent his full-time in preaching. He was well versed in classical Tamil and Telugu and worked on translation of the New Testament and in writing other books. Although no longer practising medicine Henry drove himself like his father and his health deteriorated. He was forced to go to the Nilgiris in 1854 to recuperate. Soon after their return, they lost two sons – one to cholera and the other soon after birth. Worsening health forced Henry and family to return to the States in 1857. The mission to India was uppermost in his mind and in America he soon became a valued speaker advocating for the work of the Board in India. Although he returned to India in 1861, he was unable to stay in the plains and went to the Nilgiris where he was engaged in translation and other literary work. The Henry Martyn Scudders finally returned to America in 1864 and after a short stint as a missionary in Japan spent the rest of his life as a much valued Pastor to several parishes till shortly before his death in 1895.

William Waterbury Scudder and Joseph Scudder

William, the second son of Dr. John, had been sent to America at the same time as Henry, but he was put in the care of his maternal grandmother. He was sent to Princeton for his education and theological training and returned to Ceylon where he was posted to Panditeripo in 1847. Amy, the old faithful maid was there and was a great help to Katherine (Mrs. William) and their daughter Kitty. They visited Dr. John and Mrs. Harriet in Madurai in 1849, and on the way back, Katherine died of Cholera. William continued to work for two more years but then went back to America in 1851. He and his brother, Joseph worked with the Board to create a new mission, the American Arcot Mission, headquartered in Vellore. Henry, William and Joseph were posted to this mission. William was tasked with the administration of this mission without much financial support. In fact, it was only the generous gifts of his sister, Harriet who had married a rich estate owner that allowed them to continue. A seminary to train evangelists, pastors and teachers was started and William also was in charge of visiting the numerous schools and churches throughout the district and settling numerous jealousies and disputes. He found the work increasingly tedious and tiresome and the fact that his brother Joseph had to return to America because of ill health did not make his life any easier. In 1872 after 26 years of service, he resigned from the mission and returned to America. He was the Pastor of a Church in Glastonbury, Connecticut for twelve years. This helped him with the education of his children. In 1884, he returned to India and was put in charge of the Seminary at Vellore till he retired in 1894. He died a year later.

Ezekiel Carman Scudder

1855, the year Dr. John died, the India he loved was in turmoil. The British East India Company was entering its last years and the first Revolution of Indian Independence was but two years away. Innovations, such as the railroad and the telegraph were seen as alien to the Indian culture and there was a great fear among many Indians that there would be forcible conversion to Christianity. Southern India was spared much of the turmoil of the first revolution of Independence but felt its tremors as it swept through northern and eastern India. Soon after the Revolution, Britain took over the governance of India from the East India Company by an Act of Parliament and this great land became part of the British Empire Under Queen Victoria. Her proclamation "We have neither the power nor the desire to impose our convictions on any of our subjects" was understood by the majority of Indians that the Crown would not compel Christianisation. It was to this India that Ezekiel and his younger brother Jared arrived.

The Arcot Mission assigned Ezekiel and his bride to Arni, a small town about 25km south of Vellore. He set up camp there but like his father was constantly on the move– visiting villages, preaching and establishing churches. Ezekiel was a joyful person and he was much appreciated by all he came in contact with. His audience were primarily from the low caste farm labourers where his message of love struck a chord. For thirteen years, Ezekiel travelled across the country and his health deteriorated due to recurrent attacks of dysentery and sunstroke. He returned to America and completed his training as a doctor because he had seen the medical needs of the people. He came back to Arni to continue his work as a preacher and now also as a healer. The following year, he was asked to take charge of the seminary at Vellore as William was leaving for America. The change from the isolation of Arni was welcome particularly to his wife, but Ezekiel's health continued to be bad and they asked to be relieved of their work in India. He accepted an offer from a parish in New Jersey and their home became a home away from home to all Scudder children who had to return to America for their education.

Jared Waterbury Scudder

The fifth of the sons of Dr. John and Mrs. Harriet returned to India as an ordained minister in 1855 and was posted to Chittoor about 25 km north of Vellore. Along with his wife, Julia, a major initiative in girls' education was evident as their distinct contribution. Like all Scudder men, Jared was involved in preaching in the market places of surrounding villages and a quotation from him is illuminating on what these missionaries encountered:

"In one instance, we were favoured with a contemptuous loathing, which did not hesitate to vent itself in words and gestures of no questionable import. We were treated like dogs. Personal violence alone was wanting to perfect the indignity... You get buckets full of filthy abuse poured over you until you feel yourself polluted in your entirety. Listen for half an hour or so to the biting sarcasm, pointed by obscene jests, seconded by the plaudits and withering laugh of a crowd in full sympathy with your foul-mouthed assailant..."

This was the experience of all the Scudder men as they went preaching from village to village. Their exhortations before they treated their patients in their clinics were tolerated and listened to because treatment followed. Was the fact that Silas and John II and several of the next generation of Scudders were primarily healers rather than itinerant preachers? Or was it he result of a recognition of the folly of preaching to captive audiences who would be waiting anxiously for the reward of their patient listening in the form of treatment? Jared and Julia established many small congregations in their area of work and their efforts at girls' education were well received. A particular activity was the arrangement of marriages for the girls who graduated from their school with the graduates of the Vellore Academy. Julia's health deteriorated and they had to go back to America in 1860. This time Jared with his wife's help qualified as a doctor as he had seen the need for medical help for the people. In the throes of the American Civil War, the Mission Board found it difficult to finance their return to India. A striking demonstration of the affection and high regard for them by the Church they established was the collection of Rs.1000 ($500) by their parishioners to pay for their passage back to India.

Jared was appointed in charge of the Vellore Seminary in 1894 when William went back to America. He retired from that post in 1908 at the age of 78. Little is known of the medical contributions of Jared but his most significant contribution was the coming together of the different mission affiliated churches as the South India United Church in 1901 of which he was elected the moderator in 1903. He and his brothers played a key role in the Indian missionary conferences in 1879, 1883 and 1893 which laid the groundwork for the union of the Arcot Mission of the Reformed Church in America, the Church of the Presbytery in Madras and the United Free Church of Scotland. Jared was a prolific writer and left behind many scholarly works including translations of his brother Henry's Tamil Books to English.

Little has been documented about the role of the wives of the Scudder men. Did they play only a passing supporting role in the ministry of their husbands? Jared's wife, Julia was the sister of the wife of the Governor of Georgia. She helped Jared in all his studies because of his weak eyesight. She was instrumental in the success of women's education at Chitoor and her unceasing efforts ensured adequate funds. But her influence was far greater. A quotation from a tribute by an Indian co-worker after her death in 1913, three years after Jared had passed away summarises her life beautifully:

"How many of our wives of "workers can look back to the years spent in school "under the influence of "her sweet quiet optimistic spirit and trace the result of "that influence on their lives and work. Even in her declining years when she could do little active work, her sweet cheerful uncomplaining spirit was ever a witness to what God can do in the human heart. During the last few months of her life "when she had a lot of distress and pain, no words of complaint passed her lips. "A brave cheerful spirit has passed away from our circle and has left with us all a "memory that is a benediction."

Silas Downer Scudder

The five, older Scudder brothers started as ordained missionaries and during the course of their work they decided that being a doctor would add the dimension of healing bodies and relief of pain to their work. So they decided that the two younger brothers should train as physicians from the beginning. Silas graduated and was working as an assistant to the Head of the Women's Hospital in New York when he felt compelled to return to India just in time to start the medical work of the

American Arcot Mission. He hoped to start a state–of–the–art hospital, but the Mission had no money for such a venture. He opened a dispensary with funds collected by some friends and in 1866, five years after he came to India, the Mission was able to find funds to support the medical work. He was able to save the life of the Nawab of Arcot who was bitten by a cobra and also treat a woman of the Nawab's household successfully. These established his credentials to such an extent that the government handed over the local civil hospital to Silas with a grant of half the amount they were spending and the old military barracks which was the Hospital. Silas was allowed by the Mission to train five young Indians so that they would be physician assistants. Four of them after three years of training, started work in the villages where the Mission had established churches and the fifth continued as his assistant. Silas was continuing a tradition that his father started but there was no attempt to formalise the training of Indian doctors. The hard work of Silas had established the hospital at Ranipet but it cost him his health. His younger brother, John II took over the hospital and Silas left India in 1872 and died two years later at the age of 44. But he had established the hospital as a crucial part of the work of the Arcot Mission.

John Scudder II

John, the youngest son of Dr. John and his wife Sophia Weld Scudder arrived in India in 1861 and was initially asked to help Silas with the medical work at Ranipet. In addition, he was posted to wherever the Mission felt he could serve as a missionary.

The Board was going through a period of severe financial difficulties and John took it upon himself to ask for more aid in a personal letter to the Secretary of the Board.

Unfortunately, this letter was shared with the Board who felt offended that the youngest missionary whom they considered a mere stripling dared to question them. This led to a big fight between the Board and the missionaries of the Arcot Mission, which was fought to a standstill, but resulted in a marginal increase in their salaries. John continued his work which included starting an industrial training school in Arcot and many evangelistic touring of the district. When Silas left, he was made in charge of the Ranipet Hospital. By 1875, he was the only one of the Scudder brothers in India but expected the three on furlough to return in due course. The timing of their return could never be forecast, due to their involvement in fundraising for the Board and the uncertainities of the sailing ships on which they were dependent. His nephew Harry, son of Henry Martyn Scudder a newly minted doctor, came and joined him at the Ranipet hospital in 1866. Promptly, John relocated to Vellore where it was easier to look after all the activities of the Arcot Mission. His medical practice thereafter was in the homes of patients who called him and after worship service in the many churches for which he was responsible.

Five boys were born to John and Sophia in India. Their longing for a daughter was fulfilled on December 9, 1870 by the birth of Ida Sophia Scudder, who grew up as the darling of her five brothers and competed to be their equal. The district was hit by a severe famine (1875 to 1877) and John and family were in the forefront of providing relief to the extent possible. The famine made an indelible impact on Ida as her responsibility was to tear up slices of bread for distribution to starving children. Finally, the famine was over when the rains that had failed for three years revived in October 1877. The John Scudder family returned to America after that for a well–deserved furlough that extended five years. John returned to India in 1883 and Sophia in 1884 leaving the children back for their education.

The third and fourth generation of Scudders in India

Ida Sophia Scudder of the third generation and Ida Belle Scudder of the fourth generation (daughter of John's second son Lewis) are central to the Vellore story. Harry (son of Henry Martin) Kitty, Lewis and Frances (Children of William Waterbury) Ezekiel Carman (son of Ezekiel Carman) Bessie and Julia (daughters of Jared Waterbury) and Henry and Walter (sons of John II) are the nine Scudders of the third generation of the family that served as missionaries in India between 1874 and 1936. All of them were part of the Arcot Mission and carried on the traditions established by Dr. John. In the fourth generation of the Scudder family, Galen, Beth, Ruth, Nelle, Maude, Helen and John served the Arcot Mission from 1919 to 1954. Several of them were medically trained and worked to convert the medical work at Ranipet from the abandoned barracks to the Scudder Memorial Hospital in 1925. It is surprising that none of them really got involved in the work that Ida Sophia was doing at Vellore nor did they make a significant effort to contribute to the development of medical education in India. The vision of catering to the health of the women and children and establishing a cadre devoted to their welfare that motivated Ida Sophia and the wider vision that catalysed Ida Belle apparently did not catch fire with others of the third and fourth generation. Their combined contribution to India is significant and is part of the thousand years of service by the Scudder family to India. The story of the Scudder Missionaries in India has been depicted in detail by Dorothy Scudder the wife of John Scudder who served at Ranipet Scudder Memorial Hospital from 1929 to 1935.

Selection and Training of Students in the 1950's (The Class of 1955)

The success of an institution with an avowed mission to provide education, service and research in health, in the Spirit of Christ, can be evaluated by the lifetime performance of groups of students. Chapter 2 evaluates a 60–year follow–up of the Class of 1955 and a 30–year follow–up of the Class of 1985. The Class of 1955 were privileged to complete their undergraduate training while Aunt Ida, the inspired Founder, was still a presence on the campus. The Class of 1985 was selected 25 years after Aunt Ida passed away. The majority of their teachers had direct contact and inspiration from Aunt Ida. This appendix details the process of selection of the students of the class of 1955 and briefly outlines their training as students.

The Selection

Applications were called by CMCV for admission to the MBBS course of the Madras University in January 1955, and an all–India entrance examination was held in mid–May at 13 centres distributed across India. Around 2000 aspirants had written the test. Based on their performance in the test and other admission criteria, a hundred candidates, fifty women and an equal number of men were called for four days of tests and interviews at Vellore. The candidates had to arrive by Wednesday and were accommodated at the women's and men's hostels. Although half of them would not be selected, they all had to come prepared to stay on for the classes that would start the following Monday. It was known that if any candidate was not able to travel by themselves to Vellore, they would be considered not mature enough for the medical course! No family members were visible when candidates arrived in the hostels.

As the candidates walked in to the Registrar's Office on Wednesday to get their documents checked, they were stunned by Prof. JC David, the Registrar, addressing them by their name, telling them their guardian's name and asking them how they had travelled to Vellore! Prof. JCD was a remarkable man who was able to recognise each candidate from the photo and other details in the application. His recognition of each candidate by name as they walked into his room was a feat that has not been achieved by any of his successors. Staying on campus in the hostels, the warm welcome by the senior students helped to calm down the candidates. Their first introduction to the process of selection was the Rorschach test applied by the Professor of Psychiatry on Wednesday evening. The plots were projected onto a screen separately for men and women and they had to write the first thoughts that came to mind. A review by the men around the dinner table suggested that very few of them would be selected if what they boasted they had written, was indeed, true. This was only a pilot experiment that was not repeated in subsequent years!

Two days of interviews started on Thursday early morning with a brief service in the Chapel after which the candidates were divided into small groups of eight to ten and assigned to faculty members, who spent the next two days with them as Group Observers. There were three Group Tasks, an outdoor task to bring down a drum of Kerosene (actually water!) from the two–floor high roof of the Anatomy Department building which was supposed to be on fire, an indoor task to plan a jail building for 1000 inmates and a group discussion where the topics had to be identified and discussed by the Group. There were three individual tasks, one testing manual dexterity and ability to prioritise and choose, the second test was mental concentration and meticulousness and the third to give a three–minute talk on a subject after thinking and planning for six minutes. At each task, there were several Test Observers who graded each candidate and gave a final score. The Group Observers used these tests as windows through which they could better understand the personality of the candidate.

The Group Observers also individually interviewed each candidate in their group to understand their motivation, background, why they wanted to become doctors and to assess whether their personality was suitable for undergoing training at CMCV. Their primary responsibility was to assess the suitability for training at Vellore. The Group Observers, the Test Observers and the Selection Committee had spent considerable time in retreats and workshops to prepare themselves for the interview process. The Group Observers were required to prepare an individual written report on each candidate and had to assign them a Stanine Grade from A (eminently suitable) to U (unsuitable) with 7 grades in between. A and B+ grades were rare. Most frequently given grades were B, C+ and C. The final Selection Board with the Selection Committee and all Test and Group Observers compiled the marks in the All India Entrance examination, the grades from the Test Observers and the Group Observers to arrive at a final Grade. The Selection Committee thereafter finalised the list of those selected and also prepared a wait list.

While the Selection Board and Committee were labouring to finalise the choices on Saturday the Candidates were taken in buses to view the charms of Vellore and the Hospital, a paradise that would be lost to half of them by the end of the day. Introduced to the four unique characteristics of Vellore, a temple without a Deity (now installed!), a river without water, a fort without a garrison and a police force without authority. Later, the group added two more – men without brain and women without beauty! They came back to the hostels for lunch and then most of them packed their bags ready for departure, hoping that they would be fortunate enough to unpack after the results were announced. There was a large assembly at the Sunken Garden at 4PM and the names and numbers of the fifty selected for training were announced. Several parents had turned up by the time the results were announced, thus many of the ones who had to go back had some family support.

Student days in the fifties

The next five and a half years are recollected as possibly the happiest years of their lives. Life in the hostels after they were welcomed in was congenial and the teaching, excellent. Learning Anatomy from Dr. Harsha and Dr. DL Graham was facilitated by Yogesh Pai, an alumnus who was taking a year in Anatomy to prepare to be a Surgeon. Prof. Dorothy Jefferson and Miss Marjorie van Vranken made Physiology a pleasure with newly graduated Chandrahasan Johnson (Johno) as a dynamic

Demonstrator. Biochemistry had Prof. Devadatta ably assisted by Mr. Joshua whose wife worked in the neighbouring Female Jail. A new entrant to the first year curriculum was Biostatistics and Sundar Rao a fresh Masters in the subject struggled to control a class at least half of whom were older than him, till finally a truce was signed. Unfortunately, the class learnt little statistics whose value was manifest only much later. Fortunately, by then Prof. Sundar Rao's book for medical students was available for those who needed it!

Johno was game for any mischief and one beautiful clear October Saturday, when there was a tutorial by him, half the class decided to climb Toad Hill with his tacit permission. Dr. Jefferson suddenly decided to give a surprise test to the class and found that half the class was not present, a never before occurrence. As she was expressing her annoyance and asking Johno to call people from the hostel, he handed her a pair of binoculars through which she could see the delinquents on or around the toad at the top of the hill. Another day had been declared a holiday for the students as there was a hartal in town as part of a language agitation. The class decided to cycle to Amriddhi for a day picnic in the foothills and invited Johno to be the mandated chaperone. About thirty youngsters, several with one of the girls on the carrier, left early morning on cycles hired from Thorapadi or borrowed from seniors. As the sun grew warmer, about five km on the way it suddenly struck the group that although they had a chaperone, they actually had not got permission for a picnic! The group parked near a tea shop and the two class representatives and Johno went back to meet the Principal Prof. P Kutumbiah. They found him at breakfast at the Big Bungalow. Aunt Ida, Ida B and Dr. Jefferson were also at table. When the three representatives trooped in sheepishly and said that they wanted permission for a picnic to Amriddhi, Aunt Ida immediately exclaimed, "There is a hartal today. Let us bow down and pray for the safety of the children". After the prayer by the Founder there was little the Principal could do other than warn the picnickers to return well before dark. Fortunately, the problems of the hartal were only in town and not out in the remote countryside.

Christian activities were an integral part of the life in College. Class prayers on Friday and Language group prayers on Saturday evenings were an occasion to meet together, pray and socialise. When she was in residence at Vellore once a year, Aunt Ida would invite each class to hold the Class Prayer in the Big Bungalow, her residence. Occasionally, one or two would be invited to have tea with her and Ida B before the prayers. The Student Christian Movement and the Evangelical Union offered the opportunity to learn more about Christianity from different perspectives. The weekly Bible classes by senior members of the faculty were a further opportunity to learn more about our faith. The high point of the week for those who chose to attend was the Sunday evening service at the College Chapel. The simple service as the twilight faded to darkness outside the windows left an indelible impression in all minds. The activities at the St. John's Church in the Vellore Fort were an additional source of inspiration.

The first one and a half years swept by and in December 1956 the Class of 1955 was confronted by the first University Examination in Anatomy and Physiology. Fortunately, there was no exam in Biostatistics as it was a subject taught only in forward–thinking CMCV. Otherwise, none of the class would have passed. Did they neglect Biostatistics because there was no exam? Probably.

The University had just agreed to have the theory papers to be answered at CMCV. The practical and oral examinations were held at the Madras Medical College in Madras (now Chennai). The results of the examination split the class with thirty-two clearing the examination and going on to the clinical years. The eighteen cleared at the next attempt in April 1957 and were called the B Batch.

CMCV introduced the integrated system of lectures from 1957, and 55 was the first class where each organ system was taught integrating the biology of health with the biology of disease and therapy. The first hour of each weekday was the integrated lecture at the Gallery Room at the College and then to the teaching hospital for Introduction to Clinical Work. The class was divided into groups of eight students and assigned to one of the senior professors, who taught them how to deal with individual patients and not interesting cases. Professor John S Carman, Director and pioneer in Urology, Prof. P Kutumbiah, Prof. MacPherson and Prof. P Koshy, the most senior surgeons and physicians of that time were assigned to instruct the class how to deal with sick human beings. The values they taught have continued to inspire the class till today.

The afternoons were spent learning Pharmacology, Pathology, Microbiology and Medical Jurisprudence (Forensic Medicine). Prof. JC David was our teacher in Pharmacology and his text book written along with two of his students on the faculty in Madras was the basis of what we learnt. Unfortunately, three months before the second MBBS examination, a new edition of the textbook came out which put enormous pressure on the students. The class also had to learn how to make mixtures (including writing appropriate prescriptions) ointments and emulsions – arts which are sadly lost in this era of evidence (sic) based medicine. Prof. Edward Gault headed the Pathology Department, which was growing with CK Job and Aleyamma Bhaktaviziam (MP) working with him. CJG Chacko and Adolph Walter were registrars. The teachers took infinite care to make sure that the students developed a real passion for Pathology. Ruth Myers was the Chief of Microbiology, ably assisted by Grace Koshy. Medical Jurisprudence or forensic pathology was an(orphan) ? and a lady teacher on a part–time basis read Das's textbook out loud for the hour. When it was a chapter – like rape– she considered it embarrassing,and she would turn her back to the class to read it out loud!

The thrill of real clinical work in Surgery and Medicine started after the introductory course. Students were allotted beds in the Unit they were posted and they had to work up the patients and present them to the clinician who would take us through the process of a preliminary clinical diagnosis with possible differentials and then walk us through the investigations to reach a final diagnosis. We were drilled in listening to the patient's complaints, using our eyes and hands to examine and critically evaluate what tests were essential for the diagnosis. There were opportunities to assist in ward procedures and also to assist the surgeons in theatre whereby holding a retractor, you had a front row view. The limited number of house staff meant that students were a part of patient care team.

All this fast paced intense work did not mean that there was no room for play. Apart from the hostel related activities, there were games. The annual trip to Bangalore for a weekend of competition with several teams, the intercollegiate matches especially Basketball and Hockey, the annual sports with intense inter–house competitions were all a time to relax and enjoy life. Going to Madras for major events, like the Centenary celebrations of the Madras University and to listen to Billy Graham were enjoyable interludes. The Class of 55 were able to persuade Dr. KG Koshy, the head of Community Medicine, that instead of going to Madras for a week for a first–hand look at public health in action, it would be far more educational to visit Bangalore, Mysore and Ooty to experience various programmes. A very enjoyable time was had by all but did they really learn anything? The experiment was not repeated subsequently! There were also many class picnics to Kailas mountain, French castle (there was no castle and whether the French ever went there is questionable but there was a pond for swimming), Sathannur dam which had a swimming pool and to Virinchipuram to view the magnificent temple. Twice a week, on Wednesdays and Fridays, two from the class in the first clinical year would accompany Dr. Ida B Scudder or Dr. DL graham on the roadside clinics, continuing the tradition started by Aunt Ida. Life was indeed busy and enjoyable.

Hostel life was the enjoyable crux of the College in those years. Both hostels provided the bare necessities in the room, a table and chair, a cupboard for clothes and a wooden cot. All soft furnishings and comforts were to be provided by the student. The women students were assigned three or more to a room and had common dormitories on the top floor where they slept. The men had the luxury of individual rooms in the recently completed men's hostel, the self–designated Mansion of the Gods! The hostels were self–regulated, each with a General Body overseen by an elected Speaker, as the elected General Secretary and Committee, who looked after the day–to– day running.

Miss Treva Marshall and Prof. KG Koshy were the wardens who provided supervision and guidance for life in the hostels. The main activity in the first term (June to September) was the celebration of the Hostel Day with tea in the hostel garden, an entertainment in the Assembly Hall and dinner back in the Hostel, when the opposite sex was allowed to be in the hostel till mid–night. All students and faculty with their families were invited for tea and the entertainment but for the dinner, individuals invited their special guests. Since in the Class of 55 ultimately seven married their classmates and a further twelve married another student or faculty, the importance of these social interactions can be understood. In three of the five Men's Hostel Days the class celebrated, the men students put up a stage in the vacant land between the hostel and the road to stage their play. But from the first year it rained continuously that day and at the last minute the play had to be shifted to the Assembly Hall, not a big problem because that was where the rehearsals were held, but was a major disappointment after all the hard work. Taking off from classes to work for these festivities was an enjoyable bonus!

Other major social events were the fresher's welcome dinner in the first term, the College Day, Baccalaureate and Graduation day in the second term, the final year farewell dinners in the second and third term. The weekly Sunday lunches in both the hostels were a high point. The faculty resident on campus would sign up for their family to have lunch in one of the two hostels. It was a formal sit down lunch with chicken biriyani with all trimmings followed by ice cream. This provided an opportunity for faculty student interaction and bonding. A tradition that is unfortunately no longer there.

Examinations came at regular intervals. The theory paper, long essay questions and a few short notes were tackled in the Assembly Hall at College Campus. The practical and oral examinations were in Madras. The college arranged for the women students to stay in the ladies hostels of the respective medical colleges in Madras but the men had to fend for themselves. The examinations in Pharmacology, Pathology, Microbiology and Forensic were 18 months after starting clinical years. Six months later was the Part 1 of the final examination in Ophthalmology. The class survived these tests of knowledge without too much trouble, a tribute to the skills of our teachers.

And then at the beginning of January 1959, the class entered the final year with University Examination looming in December. Three brilliant young medical teachers had joined the faculty, Hari Vaishnava, XJ Ankelesaria and FM Narielwala, who took a personal interest in preparing the students for the examination, which also prepared them to be exceptional clinicians. They supplemented the senior teachers Profs. P Kutumbiah, Philip Koshy and Kamala Vaithilingam. In surgery, Profs. Paul Brand, HS Bhatt, Ian Macpherson and Donald Hancock were the inspiration supplemented by LBM Joseph and AS Fenn who obtained their MS in surgery that year. Obstetrics and Gynaecology were the realm of Profs. Carol E Jameson, D Paranjothi and Miriam Manuel. Each student had to do three week residential posting in Medicine, Surgery and Midwifery staying overnight at the Hospital. A highlight was each student being responsible for personally attending 20 normal deliveries and submitting their detailed notes at the final examination. There were clinics in the afternoons and night and long hours spent pouring over text books and notes from lectures and clinics. All of this culminated in the theory examinations at Vellore starting on December first and practical and oral examinations a week later in Madras.

The Class of 1955 negotiated these barriers without too much trouble and by June of 1960 all were interns in the College responsible for patient care in Medicine, Surgery, Obstetrics and Community health. Once the year of Internship was over, they had to confront the wider world. Many went to work in mission hospitals while a few stayed on for a house job at CMCV and on to a postgraduate course. This was also a time when it was relatively easy to go for further training and to work in countries abroad. Thirteen of the thirty–eight 1st postgraduate degrees were obtained by training in UK or USA. Twenty 1st postgraduate degrees were from CMCV and five from other Indian institutions.

The record of accomplishments by the Class of 1955 listed at the beginning shows that the process of selection was based on suitability for training at CMCV and not purely on academic excellence from students who in general were just above average– a valuable strategy. This was coupled with rigorous in–service training in a Gurukul atmosphere on the campus with close interactions with the teachers. The record after nearly sixty years from the time they joined showed that while none of them were yet billionaires, they had lived up to the motto of the Institution and had held the CMCV flag high. They were average students but their professionalism was above average with some memorable contributions. The life and witness of one of the class Dr. Stephen Hansdak from the Santhal Tribe of Chhattisgarh is a testimony to the achievement of relevant excellence by the training at CMCV.

Author's Biography

My wife and I joined the MBBS class in the Christian Medical College Vellore in June 1955 having completed the Intermediate Course. We were both seventeen and a half years old, just enough to qualify for the medical course! We superannuated from the faculty in 1997 after about 42 years as part of the Campus Community at Vellore. We had a year and a half of study leave in Boston (1970–71) and two brief sabbaticals (1986 and 1993) while on the faculty.

My father, VM Ittyerah, obtained his MA in History and Political Science from the Madras Christian College in 1919 and joined there as a lecturer. His close friend and mentor, Mr. KC Chacko, was keen that a Christian Arts and Science College should come up in the Travancore– Cochin area (the southern half of present Kerala) as a joint venture of the main non–Catholic churches, The Malankara Jacobite Church, Mar Thoma Syrian Church and the CMS (now Church of South India, Madhya Kerala Diocese). He was able to persuade three young men, my father, Mr. CP Mathew and Mr. AM Varki to join him and start the Union Christian College as a residential Christian institution, in 1921 at Alwaye near Cochin, in North Travancore. My mother, Anna Alexander, was teaching in the Nicholson Girls High School of the Mar Thoma Church in Thiruvella. They met each other and married in early 1936. I was their first child in 1937, and I have a younger sister.

It was a privilege to grow up on the campus of the college, where my parents were the non-resident wardens, initially of the women's hostel and later of the Holland Hostel, one of the largest men's hostels on the campus. We lived in a house on the main campus, next to the Holland Hostel. My sister and I grew up in this comfortable three bedroom house till she left to join the Women's Christian College in Chennai, after completing high school and I left to join CMCV a year later in 1955. My father retired from the Union Christian College in 1955 and took over as Principal of the Mar Thoma College, run by our Church in Thiruvella.

I was privately tutored in the first grade at home and joined a primary school run by the college, as a contribution to the surrounding community, in grade two. Unfortunately, the change I noticed after my last visit to the college in 2017, the building of this school had disappeared. The next two grades I did at the nearby Settlement School, started by a few alumni of the college to help disadvantaged children. When I was ten years old and entering the fifth grade, my mother along with some of the other faculty wives, decided to revive a Christian girl's residential school, the Christava Mahilalayam, about five kilometres on the other side of the town of Alwaye. I spent a year as one of three boys in this girl's school where my mother was also teaching. At that age, it was not an enjoyable experience!

An incident in that year set the direction of my life. Our local doctor referred my mother to Vellore as he felt she should have a hysterectomy. While my parents went to Vellore, I stayed with the headmistress of the school and was very homesick. However, she came back in a few days as the doctors in Vellore decided that her heart was too weak to stand such major surgery. I now know that both decisions were wrong as she lived another forty–five years till she was ninety–one, without either a hysterectomy or major heart problems! Her vivid descriptions of Dr. Ida Scudder and other doctors of Vellore during hospitalisation motivated me and I decided I wanted to be a doctor and that I should be trained at Vellore.

At the end of the year at Mahilalayam, there was a lot of discussion at home whether I should be sent to a boarding school where my uncle was the Principal, but finally much to my relief it was decided that I would stay at home and join the St. Mary's English High School in town, commuting three kilometres each way. About ten of us boys from in and around the college walked to school every morning. We would leave home by about eight in the morning and reach school about a quarter of an hour before it started. Lunch break was from 12.30 to 1.30 and that meant running to a neighbouring house of friends of my parents' to have my packed lunch. Lunch was always either boiled egg sandwiches or bread, butter, and beef cutlets. I still prefer this for lunch, but seldom get it! After lunch, we would rush back to school to play till classes started at one thirty. At the end of the day, our group from College Hill would gather and walk back together. When the State Transport Corporation started local bus services, I was given a season ticket so that the three–kilometre walk was replaced by a ten–minute bus ride though it was not half as enjoyable as my walk.. On reaching home, I would gobble up whatever my mother had ready for tea and run off to play cricket with my friends. We enjoyed ourselves but never excelled in the game as we were only playing for fun!

In the 1940s, there was no thought of becoming professional career sportsmen, we just enjoyed.

In St. Mary's, I soon proved myself an excellent student and won a government merit scholarship of seventy–two rupees a year during my last three years in school, covering my tuition and a little towards books. They had an excellent library and I had finished most of Dickens and Scott by the time I completed school. However, the daily commute meant that I could not seriously take part in games. In the last two years of school, I had grown quite tall and used to play basketball with the college students whenever I had time in the evening as the court was next to our house on campus. I was very determined that I should become a doctor and found out that additional weightage in selection to the State Government Medical College would be given for extracurricular activities, especially if you were a member of a college team that won at least district honours. By the time I was in the School Final Class (called Sixth Form at that time, the eleventh year of school), I was playing basketball regularly with the college students, every evening when I was free.

I was expecting very good grades and a state rank in the school final examination. When the results came, while I had a First Class and was first in my school, I did not have a state rank. My father later found out that for my English second paper officially I got only four marks, although the actual mark was forty four, because the examiner who valued made a mistake in transcribing the marks. We found this out much later and did not pursue it further (I passed because I got forty out of fifty for English First Paper). In 1953, I joined the Intermediate Course in Union Christian College in the Second Group with Biology,

Physics and Chemistry as subjects, to prepare for admission two years later to Medical College.

Sixteenth of June 1953 is a day I will never forget. After passing the school final examination, I was waiting for college to open and classes to begin in the third week of June. I was a voracious reader and used this opportunity to catch up on a lot of reading. I was reading in my room when I heard the gate creak as someone opened it. I looked up and saw a vision that changed my whole life as a mother and daughter walked in. Dr. TC Thomas had just been posted as the Chief Medical Officer at the Alwaye Government Hospital. Mrs. Thomas was bringing her second daughter, Minnie, to meet my mother to request admission for her in the Second Group in College. I saw the girl with whom I decided to spend the rest of my life! She and I along with 46 others were admitted to the Second Group in College. The social customs were such that I must confess that I hardly talked to her for the next two years of college. The boys would come to class a few minutes before time. The girls in the class would wait as a group outside the ladies waiting room till the bell rang and they knew the teacher would be at the door of the class when they walked in. When the class finished, the teacher would wait for the girls to leave before leaving the class. Hardly any chance for conversation! I wonder if these old world traditions still continue at Alwaye?

Two years in the Intermediate Class in Group Two passed quickly. There were many competitive tests with prizes in college and I competed, usually successfully, for most of them. I even won a prize for Malayalam short story writing, probably reflecting the lack of competition! An interesting experience was in my second year when the two pastors of my Church who were students in my class, while they were also the pastors to the college and to the town of Alwaye, suggested to my father that I should not take part in the annual Bible knowledge competitive examination in the college as they were afraid I would come first. My father would not interfere and I am afraid the two pastors decided not to compete! I was a member of the college basketball team and we became the Divisional Intercollegiate champions, although we lost to St. Berchman's College, Chenganassery at the Interdivisional stage.

My two years as a student of the Intermediate Class, staying at home, in the college founded by my father were very enjoyable. The problems of a faculty child caught up with me when I decided to stand for election for College Union Secretary in the second year. I am afraid the students ganged up on me to make sure that a faculty child was not elected. I did well in studies, passing the Intermediate University Examination in the First Class, with state rank in the Group Two subjects. Although a seat in the State Medical College in Trivandrum was certain, I was determined that I should gain admission to the Christian Medical College Vellore. As soon as the university examination was over, my diligent preparation for admission to Vellore started. After the written entrance test, I was sure I had done very well and would be called for the interview. What I was concerned about most was whether my classmate Minnie would also be called as I wanted her to continue to be my classmate, hopefully to become my lifemate, although we had not talked to each other in class for two years!

During the first week of June 1955, we heard from CMC that both were called for the selection interview scheduled for the last week of the month. We reached Vellore on a Wednesday and the interview started that evening with psychological tests involving Rorschach plots. We were never told what these tests revealed! The detailed interviews and tests kept us busy on Thursday and Friday, and we were taken for visits to the fort and the hospital on Saturday morning, while the selection committee met. The afternoon was spent packing our bags to go home in case we were not selected when the results were announced in the Sunken Garden at college in the evening that. Minnie and I were among the fifty students selected.

The four and a half years as a student on the Vellore campus passed all too quickly. I did well academically, graduating with the best outgoing student Gold Medal instituted in memory of Dr. JC David's mother. The college started giving certificates of merit for academic excellence only when I was in the final year and instituted a gold medal for the best student in general medicine that year. There were no other prizes for academic excellence at that time unlike the current situation. I was placed in the First Class and first rank in the University in the final MBBS examination, the second student to do so, after Khurshid Jeejeebhoy two years earlier. Internship was completed by January 1961 and I joined as Senior House Surgeon for a year to qualify for admission for the Postgraduate course in General Medicine. Midway through the year, I was told by Mrs. Naomi Carman, the then Treasurer that I had to fulfil a two-year service obligation for the scholarship I received during the last three years of the MBBS course, before I could join postgraduate training. I had assumed that the scholarships were in recognition of my academic merit and had not realised there was a price to pay! The scholarships were more than welcome as my father had retired and I had no regrets about working for two years for the Institution as I had already decided that I would like to spend my working life there.

One year of the service obligation was completed serving as a Research Fellow in the Wellcome Research Unit, leading a field team studying an epidemic of Tropical Sprue, staying in Wandiwash about eighty kilometres to the southeast of Vellore. Selwyn Baker, Professor of Medicine and Head of Medicine Unit 1, had obtained a grant from the Wellcome Trust to study this epidemic. The team stayed in a large shed at the Mission Compound in Wandiwash and surveyed the surrounding villages, identifying and treating patients affected in the epidemic and trying to study the epidemiology and microbiology of the illness to understand its aetiology. The seriously ill and those who we felt merited further investigation were sent to Vellore for admission in the metabolic ward of the Wellcome Unit for detailed study. We would stay in the field for the week and come back to Vellore on Saturday evening and return Sunday evening. On the weekend, I would be in the ward looking after the patients referred from the field and confirming that they had malabsorption. This was my introduction to research.

I was fortunate that it involved studying an epidemic for which we set up a field laboratory to confirm that patients had malabsorption of nutrients. I, therefore, gained experience in field work, patient care and in supervising a laboratory. This work was presented by me at the Joint Annual Conference of the Association of Physicians of India in January 1962 at Indore. At the end of my presentation, Prof. PN Chuttani, the then President of the Indian Society of Gastroenterology, who had chaired the session, invited me to become a member of the Society, just a year after completing Internship. I was able to join since the

Hospital paid the annual subscription! I will be completing 62 years as a member of the Indian Society of Gastroenterology by January 2024. I served six years as the Secretary (1974 to 80) and was President of the Society in 1981.

The Wellcome Research Unit was started by Selwyn Baker who joined the faculty of CMC in 1955 after working for a year with Prof. John Dacie at the Royal Postgraduate Medical School, London UK. He joined Prof. P Kutumbiah in Medicine Unit 1 and when Prof. Kutumbiah retired became head of Medicine Unit 1 in 1958. Selwyn arrived in Vellore with a modest research grant from the Wellcome Trust to study Nutritional Megaloblastic Anaemia. By 1957, he showed that megaloblastic anaemia in non–pregnant adults in and around Vellore was almost invariably associated with chronic diarrhoea and malabsorption. The Wellcome Trust then provided him funds to build a Metabolic Ward with a laboratory in the basement to take this interesting observation further. The Ward and the Wellcome basement laboratory were adjacent to the Department of Neurological Sciences and shared facilities with Neurochemistry. The Ward had ten metabolic study beds and laboratory facilities were available for Haematology and Biochemical work in the basement.

In the mid nineteen–sixties, the Research Corporation in New York gave a large grant to Vellore to build a suitable memorial to Robert Ramapatanam Williams who patented the synthesis of Vitamin B1. The income from this patent was the major funding for the Research Corporation. CMCV put up the Williams Research Building on the Hospital campus to commemorate the birth of Dr. Williams to missionary parents in Ramapatanam in Andhra Pradesh. This building spread over six floors and a basement provided laboratory space for the Nutrition Research group under the leadership of Prof. Sheila

Pereira, the Neurobiochemistry group with Prof. BK Bachawat and the Wellcome Research Unit. The building had two floors for an animal house, two and a half floors for laboratories, a library and conference room. The ground floor connected with W ward and provided additional space for metabolic beds for research and the basement had cold and deep freeze rooms and an isotope laboratory and connected with the original Wellcome basement. Selwyn Baker was responsible for planning and running this facility. Two senior faculty working with Selwyn in the Research team were AN Radhakrishnan, Professor of Biochemistry and Prema Bhat, Professor of Microbiology. The research unit was as a multidisciplinary research team, in which I was responsible for the clinical and field research components.

In August 1962, I completed a year as Research Fellow and joined back to complete my interrupted House Surgeon year. I completed the six months as a Casualty Medical Officer as it gave me ample time to continue my work at Wandiwash in which I had become totally involved. In those years, the casualty functioned from 11.00 AM to 7.00 AM the next day. There were three Casualty Medical Officers. One would be on call 11.00 AM to 8.00 PM, the next would take over for the 8.00 PM to

7.00 AM shift and would be off till the 11.00 AM shift on the following day. This, essentially meant that, the person was off duty for 28 hours before they had to start duty again. The work in casualty was not heavy and all patients admitted to the six beds in Casualty were the responsibility of the Unit they were admitted under. The duties as Casualty Medical Officer allowed me to have two days out of three when I could do what I was interested in. In fact, most Casualty Medical officers in those days were faculty wives who were looking for light duty! It gave me ample time to supervise and visit the field where we were studying diarrhoeal diseases.

I was prepared to do one more year as Research Fellow with Selwyn to complete my service obligation but the faculty of the Division of Medicine insisted that I should join the MD General Medicine programme in April 1963, without serving the second year of obligation so I could join the faculty without further delay. I am afraid that I never formally completed the second year of service obligation for the scholarship although I spent the rest of my professional life at CMCV! The MD General Medicine programme in April 1963, had two other students along with me, Thomas Kuruvilla and S Krishnaswamy, They had applied for the surgical postgraduate course unsuccessfully and were then offered seats in the MD programme as I was the only applicant for MD and there were four seats! For the first time in over ten years, more than one candidate was registered for the MD. There was no formal training or classes and we learnt by being responsible for the patients in our care and discussions during rounds. CK Eapen (1961) and my classmate VX Mathew (1962) were the lone MD students from earlier years. I should have joined the course with VX but was delayed due to the year I spent as Research Fellow in Wandiwash. Any regrets about this delay? Absolutely not, that was the year that dictated the course of my professional career. I continued to be responsible for the field research programme of the Wellcome Unit during the time I was a postgraduate student studying for the MD irrespective of my other postings. Saturday afternoons and Sundays when not on call, was time for field work.

Minnie and I had decided that we should spend the rest of our lives together and we were married in April 1962. We began our life together in Room 116 on the ground floor of what was then the new MIQ. We graduated to a Harley Street house and then to a one bedroom flat in the multiplex. I got a severe attack of Chickenpox when we were staying in the multiplex and developed an allergic eye problem, just six months before the MD examination. It was impossible to follow the instructions of the Ophthalmologists not to read at that time, but by God's grace I recovered fully. The theory and practical examination for the MD in 1965 were in Chennai and I was successful at the first attempt. The theory examination was on Monday, Tuesday and Wednesday and the Practical and viva on Thursday. At the end of the Viva Voce, I was told that I was successful although the result would officially come much later.

Minnie and I were clear that our future was at CMC Vellore and that we would like to spend our life of service there, if possible. She had already completed two years of the three–year course leading to MD in Pathology. It was her salary as Demonstrator in Pathology that kept us going while I was earning ninety rupees a month as an MD trainee. The morning after the Viva, I met Dr. Chandy at the Neurology Office. He was the Principal and responsible for the appointment of new junior faculty. He asked only one question, 'Does Baker have the money to pay for you in his special fund?' On getting an affirmative answer he asked me to join immediately as Junior Lecturer Medicine (Research) in Medicine Unit 1. The appointment order came in due course after the results were officially announced! What (That) was the significance of my salary coming from a Special Fund and of the "(Research)" notification on my appointment order?

All faculty appointments are usually made against available cadre supported by the maintenance budget of the Institution, implying that the position is permanent. The Wellcome Research Unit was the first large department where the entire staff, faculty and others, except the Head of Unit, were paid from Research Special Funds. It was originally attached to Medicine Unit 1 and started by Selwyn Baker, Professor of Medicine who was the Head of both. The research grants were time bound and it was the responsibility of the Principal Investigator (the Head of Unit) to ensure availability of funds so that good scientists would be prepared to join and work in such units on a long–term basis rather than grant to grant. The Institution made provision for paying Provident Fund, Gratuity, Pension and other benefits, including medical privileges for employees, from Special Funds. However, there was always the uncertainty regarding the permanence of the appointment and all appointments were for a fixed term. All Special Fund appointment orders had an overprint in large letters "This is a Special Fund Appointment and it will be valid only as long as funds are available". I was the first to be offered an open ended Special Fund faculty appointment and to be confirmed and promoted on that. Even my appointment order as Professor of Gastroenterology and Medicine in 1973 had this superscript.

Minnie obtained MD in Pathology in 1966 and was appointed to the faculty of the Department of Pathology. We lived on the hospital campus starting in a single room in the Men Internes Quarters, then to a Harley Street one–bedroom house,then a flat in the multiplex followed by a two–bedroom quadruplex and finally a large three bedroom flat in Shanthi Illam. I was sad when many years later I was responsible for knocking down all these buildings for putting up high rise accommodation for the staff to build the Ida Scudder Centenary block. Staying in the hospital campus allowed coming home for lunch and being constantly available for your patients when emergency arose. Night rounds were the norm for consultants who stayed in the hospital. When I shifted to the College Campus, it was the norm to visit the ward as the last port of call before going home, usually late in the evening, to make sure your patients were all right and to try and pre-empt night calls. However, emergencies called us back many nights.

I continued my field work on the epidemiology of diarrhoeal diseases in addition to the full clinical and teaching load as a Research Faculty in Medicine Unit 1. We maintained a field team and I would be in the field at least one day in the week. In order to understand the epidemiology of diarrhoeal diseases in the community, long-term surveillance was initiated in Kammasamudram village about twenty kilometres south of the College Campus. I registered for a PhD in the Faculty of Medicine of the then Madras University and submitted my thesis on the Epidemiology of Diarrhoeal Diseases in southern India just before leaving for eighteen months study leave in March 1970. During my study leave, I was Senior Research Associate with Prof. RM Donaldson at the Boston University School of Medicine, Boston Massachusetts, USA. Bob's Department of Gastroenterology was considered one of the premier departments in the USA at that time. Minnie also joined this group, working with Jerry Trier in Electron Microscopy. We enjoyed the eighteen-month experience and I published three papers and Minnie two papers based on our research in Boston. Our fellowship initially was for a year but the Wellcome Trust extended it for us to complete the work we had started. We were offered faculty positions at Boston University at the end of one year but we were clear that we wanted to spend the rest of our lives at Vellore and declined the offers with our heartfelt thanks. The savings from our fellowships enabled us to buy a Premier Padmini car on our return so that we could stay on the College Campus where we shifted to, soon after our return from study leave. We used this car for nearly sixteen years and sold it for more than we paid for it when we left for a sabbatical in 1986!

I was promoted to Associate Professor of Medicine and Gastroenterology with effect from April 1971 in (to) 1975. Why this delay? Prof. N Madanagopal the Head of the Department of Gastrointestinal Sciences at the Madras Medical College and the Madras General Hospital had returned to India after training in Gastroenterology in the UK in 1965. The Government posted him as the Assistant to Prof. Rathinavelu Subramaniam in his Medical Unit. In fact, Madan was the Medical Registrar in charge of the MD General Medicine examination in April 1965 when I appeared. It was his decision that patients for the clinical examination would be brought from other hospitals and not from the Madras General Hospital that created an even field, with the local students being as ignorant as me, of the clinical details when allotted the cases at the clinical exam. All of us had to depend on history taking and clinical skills to discuss and present the case. I was the only successful candidate from the twenty who took the clinical examination that day! I have always been grateful to Madan for his scrupulous honesty in conducting that examination. Madan and I became good friends and we were keen that we should start the DM course in Gastroenterology at the same time in Vellore and Madras. The DM Gastroenterology training programme was already in place at the All India Institute of Medical Sciences, New Delhi (AIIMS) and the Post Graduate Institute of Medical Education and Research at Chandigarh,

(PGIMER). Both these were autonomous Central Government Institutions and the red tape involved in starting a new special postgraduate course was much less for them compared to Departments affiliated to a State University. Since both of us only had MD in General Medicine from the Madras University and no degree in Gastroenterology, the University took its time to accept our experience in Departments of Gastroenterology outside India before approving the start of the course.

The first examination for the DM programme was in 1976 for the first candidate from Madras Medical College and the first candidate from Vellore appeared in 1979. George Kurien joined the Gastroenterology Clinic in 1976 and was the first recipient of DM Gastroenterology from Vellore. David Rolston was the second successful candidate the next year. George and David joined the faculty of the unit. We had obtained a forward– viewing ACMI gastro–duodenoscope in 1974 through a grant to study gastric physiology in iron deficiency anaemia. This acquisition helped us to develop a very busy gastrointestinal endoscopy diagnostic service, one of the first in India. Further scopes and accessories were purchased from the money earned by the endoscopy service. When we started in 1974, Olympus was not established in India but by 1979 the company was well established and ours was the first Unit to have a full diagnostic and therapeutic endoscopy service. I must give full credit to my clinical colleagues in Gastroenterology, George Kurien, David Rolston, BS Ramakrishna and Ashok Chacko for developing this excellent service. I gave them access to funds and freedom to make all professional decisions to develop the Gastroenterology services. The Institution allowed us to operate the endoscopy service initially as a special fund operation. All the fees charged for endoscopy were credited to an Endoscopy special Fund. All expenses –the salaries of three consultants, nurses and technician as well as the cost of repairs and replacement of the scopes were debited to the fund. The endoscopy service provided ample funds for the development of the Gastroenterology and Hepatology Department. Seven years after I started a Gastroenterology Clinic in 1972, the service was fully established and more than earning its keep. The Institution then approved the GE clinic becoming a fully budgeted Gastroenterology and Hepatology Department.

Consequent to the big strike in 1975, Selwyn Baker was constrained to leave the Institution. He started his career at Vellore in 1955 as a missionary supported by the Church Missionary Society, but from 1972 he held a position in the World Health Organisation (WHO) and his salary was paid by the Wellcome Trust through a special grant to the WHO. At the end of the 1975 strike, one of the major fallouts was that the state authorities pressurised the WHO to abolish the post occupied by Selwyn. The WHO, being a multilateral organisation required the permission of the Government to maintain their staff in India. The State Government saw this as an ideal opportunity to pay back CMCV for their steadfast resistance to the Government's proposals for compromise during the strike. Selwyn had to resign and leave Vellore after twenty–one years of service. In a few months, Selwyn found a position as Professor of Gastroenterology at the University of Winnipeg in Manitoba, Canada.

At the same time, two other Senior Faculty of the Wellcome Research Unit, Dr. AN Radhakrishnan, Professor of Biochemistry and Dr. Mrs. Prema Bhat, Professor of Microbiology also resigned and relocated to Hyderabad and Bangalore respectively. I was the sole remaining Faculty in the Unit which had about ten skilled technicians in Biochemistry, Microbiology, Haematology and field work. The problems confronting me were compounded by the Wellcome Trust informing them that their support to Vellore actually was only a personal grant to Selwyn and would not be continued. They were prepared to give approximately Ninety Thousand Pounds to pay termination benefits to all the staff employed in the unit, which included me. The then Deputy Director of the Wellcome Trust was sent to Vellore to sort all this out.

I must pay a tribute to Dr. LBM Joseph, the Director of CMCV and his administrative colleagues who were very supportive at this time. I was able to convince the administration based on the record of the Gastroenterology Clinic for the preceding four years, that a new Department of Gastroenterology would be a viable proposition. A budget was approved for the Gastroenterology Department. Salaries of faculty including mine were paid from the Endoscopy special fund to which all the receipts from endoscopies were credited. The future of the Wellcome Research Unit was still uncertain.

I obtained funds from the British Council to attend a one-week course on Paediatric Gastroenterology in the UK in early 1976 and used the opportunity to have detailed discussions with Dr. Bridget M. Ogilvie, the then Director of the Wellcome Trust and Prof. Gordon Smith, Director of the London School of Hygiene and Tropical Medicine, one of the Trustees of the Wellcome Trust. I was able to convince them that it would be a pity to disband the very valuable resource of skilled technologists and a well-equipped metabolic laboratory built over twenty years with the Trust support when there were so many priorities including Tropical Sprue that required further research. The research plans outlined for the next three years were accepted and modest support for three years' work was granted. It was also agreed that if the work was satisfactory, the Trust would make the Vellore Unit one of the Wellcome Trust Tropical Disease Research Units. There were three such Units at that time in Nairobi, Jamaica and Bangkok. The Trust and the Vellore Administration accepted this plan of action.

Establishing a new clinical service, the Gastroenterology Unit, continuing the research activities of the Wellcome Unit and raising additional funds to sustain the research momentum were all the responsibilities I had accepted to look after the myriad legal problems that confronted the Institution after the 1975 seventy day strike. These were the challenges I had to successfully overcome during the latter half of the 1970s. I was able to persuade Peter Hill, a missionary working in the Clinical Biochemistry Department to relocate to the Wellcome Unit. It was necessary to convince the administration that this would be in the best interest of the Institution and of Kanagasabapathy, the other Clinical Biochemist in the Institution. Jasper Daniel and Deva Prasanna Rajan, both with MSc in Microbiology, working in the service department in the Hospital agreed to transfer themselves to the Unit on my assurance that they would be able to register for a Doctoral programme in Microbiology. I was able to persuade the University to accept my credentials to be their Supervisor because of my PhD in the Faculty of Medicine and my publications. Both of them successfully obtained their doctoral degree, did excellent research and also served the Institution in administrative capacities.

Jasper Daniel was a very successful General Superintendent of the Institution for almost 8 years. Rajan served as a Deputy Director with distinction.

Another critical addition to the department was Dr. KA Balasubramaniam, a Research Biochemist. We knew that Peter Hill would have to return to the UK shortly as his children were reaching the age when they would have to join schools there. Balu had done his PhD with Prof. Bachawath in the Neurochemistry Unit earlier and had done Post–Doctoral fellowships in the USA. His home was in Vellore and we were able to persuade him to join the research team. He proved to be a valuable addition and continued to be responsible for the Unit's research when Minnie and I superannuated in 1997.

In 1972, shortly after my return from study leave, one of my patients was the son of the leading trial lawyer in Chennai. His mother already was LBM's patient and so the Institution had a close relationship with the family. In all the legal hassles, we were represented by the firm King and Partridge in Madras. Our point of contact was a partner in the firm Mr. C Doraiswamy (CD) and his junior in 1975 was Mr. S Ramasubramaniam (SRS). Two other younger advocates, Mr. Krishna Srinivasan and Mr. Sanjay Mohan had just joined the firm. This legal team developed a close relationship with the Institution. I was the liaison between this legal team and CMCV Administration. During the 1975 seventy day strike, I visited Chennai at least fifty times for legal purposes. Even after the strike was over several hours each week were devoted to working with the personnel office at Vellore and with CD and SRS in Chennai or attending court when our cases were being heard.

By 1977, I ended up with what were three full-time responsibilities. The nurturing and development of the Clinical Gastroenterology Department, guiding the multidisciplinary research team in the Wellcome Research Unit to ensure optimum productivity and the responsibility for all the legal problems that resulted for the Institution from the seventy day strike. I was physically present in court while the lengthy legal process consequent to the strike wound its way through the courts to the Honourable Supreme Court of India and was then referred to arbitration by a retired Supreme Court Judge. The Arbitrator's award was finally given in 1989 settling the legal problems that troubled us for nearly fifteen years. My full involvement in Clinical Gastroenterology continued till George Kurien, the first DM in Gastroenterology from Vellore was recognised as Professor of Gastroenterology. When he was joined by David Rolston, Ashok Chacko and BS Ramakrishna,with all my students for gastroenterology, I could safely withdraw myself completely from the Department. By that time I had accepted additional responsibilities and was the Medical Superintendent of the Hospital from 1988.

The Wellcome Trust provided funds for a year's sabbatical for Minnie and me in 1986. Minnie chose to work with Prof. Whitehead at the Flinders University in Adelaide and I was with Prof. Derek Rowley at the Adelaide University. Our daughter Anila went with us and we had a memorable year professionally, socially and culturally. What made our sabbatical particularly enjoyable were our classmates Dora and Mohan Rao who had emigrated to Adelaide. Their family welcomed us with open arms and helped to make our stay memorable. The freedom from routine responsibilities and being able to devote our time fully to research made this year professionally very rewarding.

I was able to establish a rat model of acute diarrhoea, which established that the mechanism of pathogenesis of acute diarrhoea in adults postulated by us could be replicated in an animal model.

LBM Joseph completed a second term as Director of CMC in 1987, and I knew that the Selection Committee for the next Director was likely to consider my name as a potential candidate for the responsibility. I therefore left a detailed letter with LBM addressed confidentially to the Chair of the Selection Committee, explaining that this letter was left with the Director in case they wanted to contact me during my sabbatical. In the letter, I explained in detail why I felt not yet ready to be considered for the post of Director of CMC at that point in time. I enthusiastically suggested Benjie Pulimood as the next Director whom I would wholeheartedly support and work with. The Committee read my letter and did not call me in Australia!

I had accepted the responsibility of being the Secretary of the Council in September 1984. The office of the Council Secretary has no administrative responsibilities but is the liaison between the Institution and the Council. The Council Secretary is a member of all the standing committees of the Institution including the Selection Committees and the Administrative Committee with the mandate to ensure that Council policies and decisions are fully carried out. The Council Secretary also has the responsibility to ensure that the views of the Director and his team are clearly enunciated to the Executive Committee and the Council. His office is responsible to ensure that all the paperwork for the Council is meticulously prepared and in a timely fashion and to do all that is necessary for the smooth conduct of the Executive and Council meetings. I carried out this responsibility along with all my other work for the next six years.

All this was possible because Minnie was prepared to move full-time to the Unit and assume several responsibilities in addition to full-time research. She applied for and was appointed as the first Career Research Professor, an avenue that was created by Council as part of its commitment to spend one-third of one percent of the maintenance budget on research. In addition to teaching Forensic Pathology to the undergraduate medical students, she took Gastrointestinal Pathology as her special area of interest. She continued to help the Pathology Department by reporting all GI surgical specimens and teaching GI Pathology to undergraduate and postgraduate students.

Benjamin Pulimood, Professor of Medicine and Head of Medicine Unit 1 was appointed as the Director in March 1987 for a seven year term. Dr. LBM Joseph had a year to complete before he attained the age of superannuation, and he accepted a year of deputation to the Christian Medical College Ludhiana as Professor of Surgery. Soon after my return from the sabbatical in Adelaide in April 1987, Benjie requested that I accept the responsibility of technology planning and development for the Institution. During the second term of LBM as Director, the Institution was in the doldrums due to the inattention of the then MS and the lack of investment in capital development. At my request, Dr.Pulimood formed a Technology Planning and Development Committee consisting of me as Chair and Dr. AS Kanagasabapathy, Professor of Clinical Biochemistry as member. This was a two- member only Committee as it gave us the freedom to make decisions and act fast. In one month, the two of us visited every Department and Unit in the Institution and discussed their future development plans in meetings where all the medical and technical personnel of the Department was present. We were able to finalise the technology upgradation requirements of each group and also able to determine from where funds would be available. In many instances, we were able to persuade the Unit to utilise funds available in their special funds to get the new equipment, ensuring that the additional income from the new facilities were also used to replenish the special funds. The Institution availed a loan of eight crore Rupees from the Industrial Development Bank of India to finance development.

The Director requested me to accept the responsibility of Medical Superintendent (MS) of the Hospital in 1988. I was concerned from the time I returned from my sabbatical that the Institution appeared to be in the doldrums and was going on its reputation and past glory with very little dynamic development. I accepted the challenge of being the MS since Benjie agreed to give me a free hand in developing the Institution with the provision that at any time he felt that I was unrealistically overenthusiastic, he could request my resignation from the MS post! I got several dynamic faculty to work with me: Dr. Bannerjea Jesudason as Deputy Medical Superintendent and Dr. Ganesh Gopalakrishnan for the Operation Theatres and Dr. Punnoose Mathew in charge of patient relations and Finance as Deputy Medical Superintendants. Very quickly, we established well– that if you came with a problem to the MS Office, it would be solved before the end of the day or you would be given a plan of action if it took longer. The MS Office became a dynamic problem solving and planning hub for the entire hospital. We reorganised the entire outpatient operation. The work of the Operation Theatres was streamlined, leading to greater efficiency and more rapid patient turnover. The MS office was established as the centre for developmental planning of clinical services. We were able to make the Hospital ready for the twenty–first century.

Benjamin Pulimood's term as Director was to be completed in March 1994 and the Council requested me in January 1994 to be the next Director, even though I would be superannuating after three and a half years in September 1997. I accepted this request, realising that I would have to work extra hard to accomplish my plans for the Institution in three and a half years. It was my constant prayer that God in His mercy would give me the wisdom and energy to accomplish what I saw as His plans for the Institution. The details of what was done in this short tenure are described in detail elsewhere and it is enough to say that I was content with what I was enabled to achieve. More than anything else, I was grateful that I earned the confidence and love of all the staff (except those I had to discipline!). I superannuated on September 26, 1997 handing over the institution to my successor. It was good to come back to Vellore for the centenary celebrations in December 2000 and see how well the Institution was doing.

The International Center for Diarrhoeal Disease Research, Dhaka, Bangladesh, offered me the position of Associate Director in charge of their Laboratory Sciences section for a three–year term from January 1998. This was an institution I was familiar with as I had served on their Board of Directors for six years till 1993. I served them for three years till December 2000 and came back to Delhi to serve as Senior Technical Adviser to the National AIDS Control Programme for a year. I relocated to Chennai (former Madras) in January 2002 and was appointed as the ICMR Chair in Epidemiology till I completed seventy years of age in 2007. I was attached to the ICMR National Institute of Epidemiology in Chennai and enjoyed this opportunity to supervise several young scientists starting their research career. We purchased a new flat in central Chennai (Chetpet) and our daughter and family had their home about a kilometre away. Minnie was appointed as an Indian National Science Academy Senior Scientist. We settled down to enjoy our retired life.

I have often felt that "retire" should actually be spelt 'retyre' as this is an opportunity to use your talents and skills in a new venture with renewed energy and vision. I have been particularly blessed to be associated with mentoring young scientists, at the National Institute of Epidemiology and in other institutions in Chennai. This has enabled me to learn about areas of medicine I had not been particularly exposed to in my career. The recent pandemic of corona virus infection has been a particularly challenging opportunity. Serving on the Ethics and Scientific Advisory Committees of the Cancer Institute in Adyar has enabled me to learn a whole new chapter in science.

I started writing these memoirs in 2021 and most of it has been written during the pandemic. We have all survived the pandemic and the world has changed. We now have to be engaged in rebuilding the new world. It is fitting to conclude with a prayer by Aunt Ida which I found among the papers in the Big Bunglow many years ago.

"May we be in such close relationship with the Father and each other that we may work together in the common round of daily tasks, That our tasks may be glorified and our work transfigured, as we see it in the light of Thy countenance.

Help us to take Thy son as the Living Partner in every act of life, make our lives become gardens of spiritual loveliness with no empty desert places. May we hear Thy voice, Help us to forgive as Thou hast forgiven us.

May Thy voice be fresh and new to us today, speak to us of Thine overflowing goodness as we listen.

Where there is suffering and sorrow may we feel Thy healing hand.

Hospital, friends, doctors, nurses, call from us the best that is in us.

When special burdens come of sickness or sorrow, give us Thy especial help and grace, Give us faith to trust Thee with our all.

Photographs

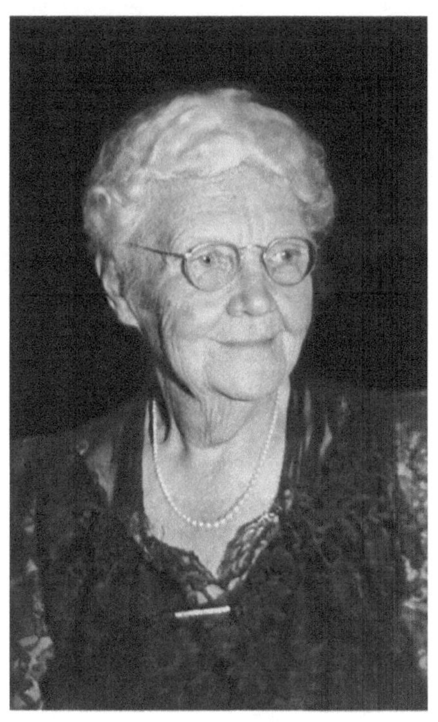

Dr. Ida Scudder

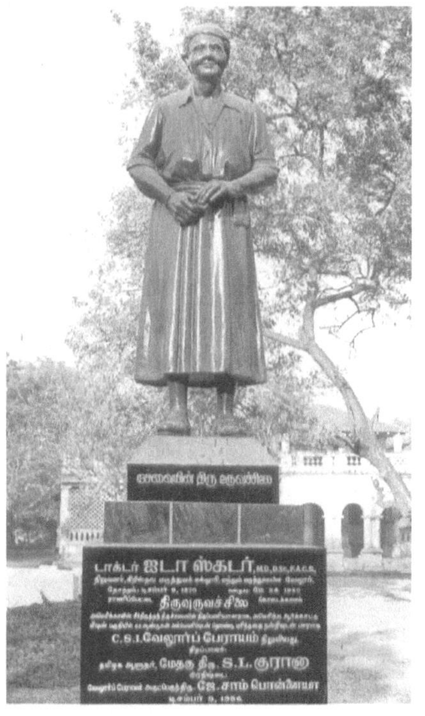

Aunt Ida's statue in town put up after her death since she refused to have one while she was alive

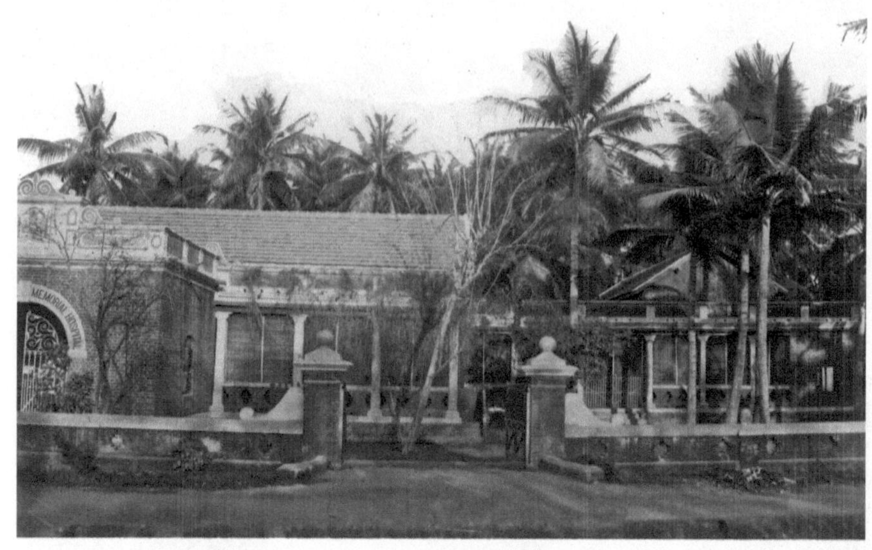

Schell Hospital Building where it all started

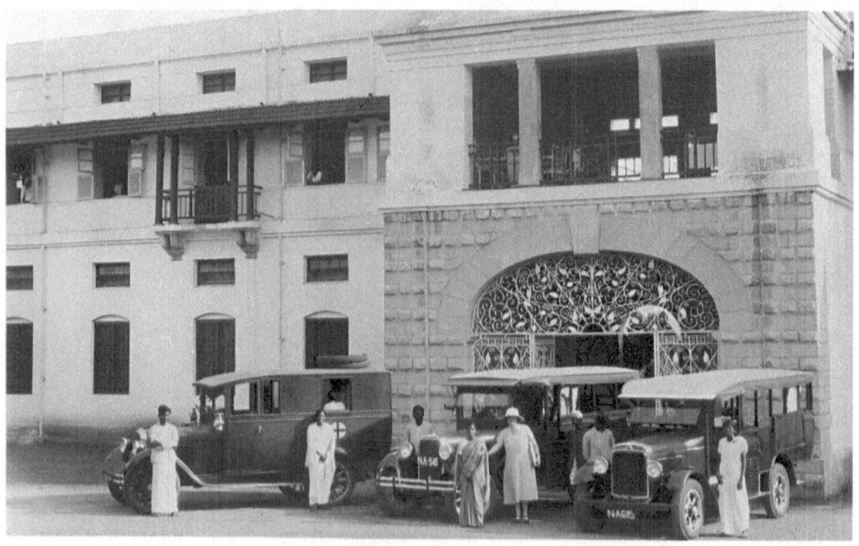

Ambulance ready to start out to their three roadside clinics

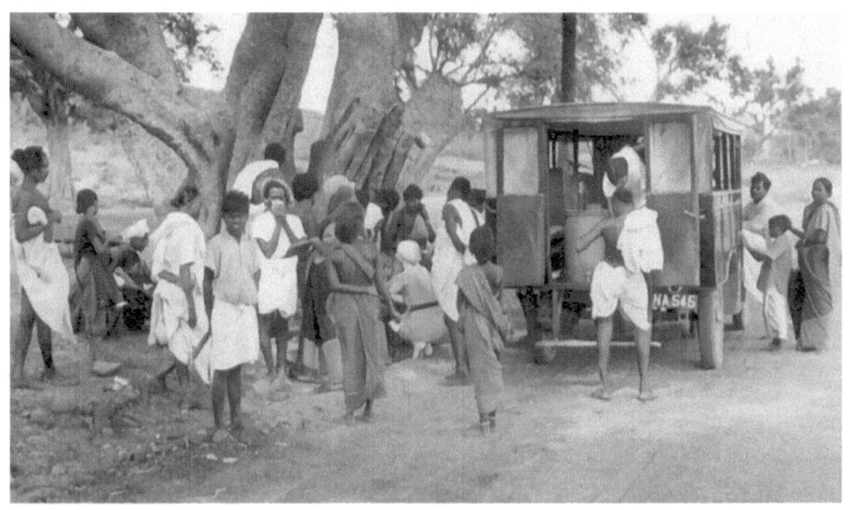

Roadside Clinic, Chittoor

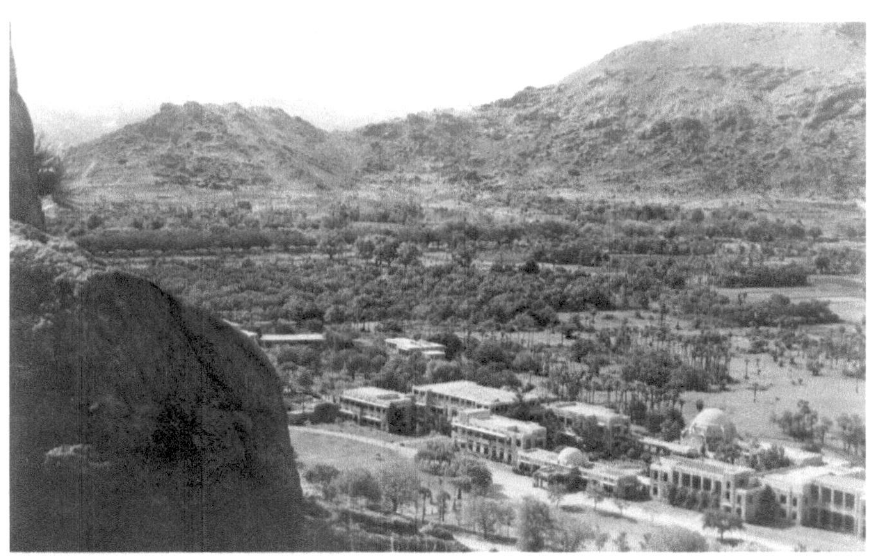

The college surrounded by hills

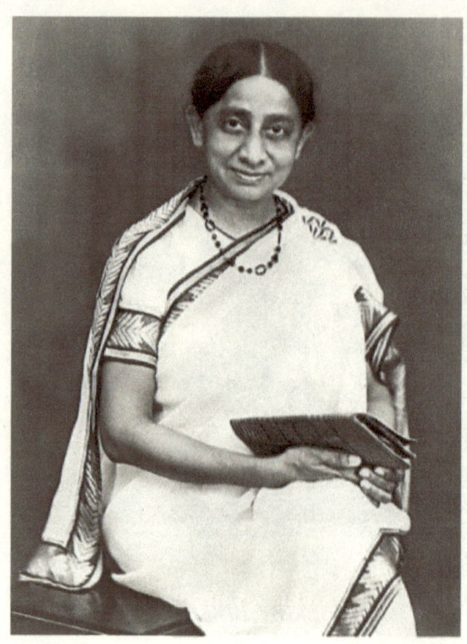

Dr. Hilda Lazarus

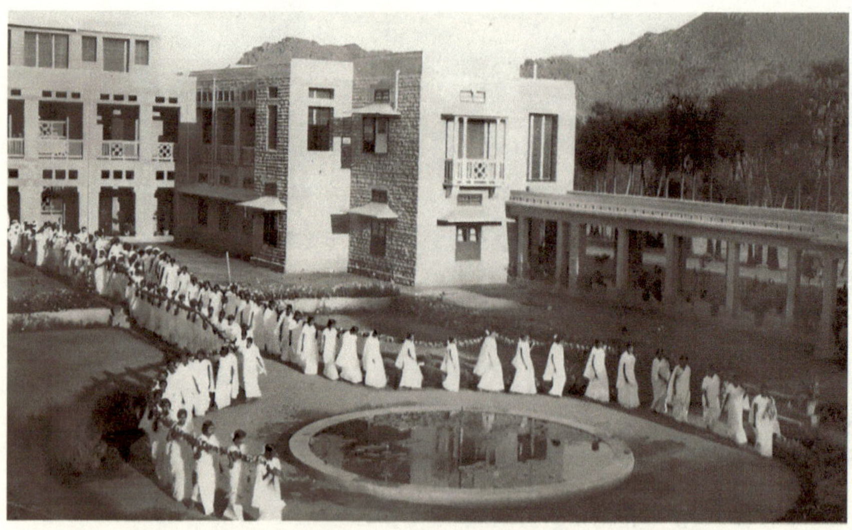

*First LMP commencement at College Hill
(Sunken Garden) graduating class 1934*

May we be in such close relationship with the Father and each other that we may work together in the common round of daily tasks, that ~~we may~~ our tasks may be glorified and our work transfigured, as we see it in the light of Thy countenance

Help us to take Thy Son as the Living Partner in every act of life

Make our lives become gardens of spiritual loveliness. With no empty desert places

May we hear Thy voice

Help us to forgive as thou hast forgiven us

Aunt Ida's handwritten prayer

May thy voice be fresh and new to us today.

Speak to us of thine overflowing goodness as we listen

Where there is suffering and sorrow may we feel Thy healing hand.

Hospital   Friends
Doctors
Nurses

Call from us the best that is in us

When special burdens come of sickness or sorrow give us thy especial help & grace

Give us faith to trust thee with our all

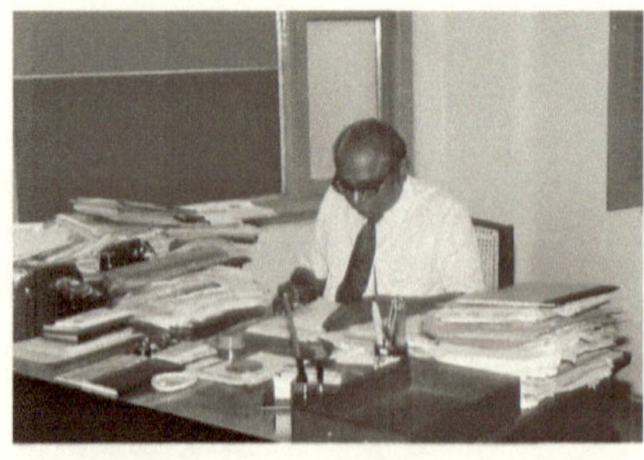

Dr. LBM Joseph at Director's Office

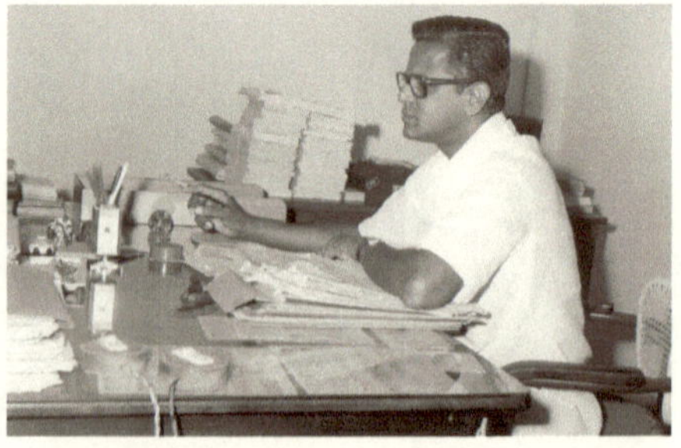

Dr. Pulimood at Principal's Office

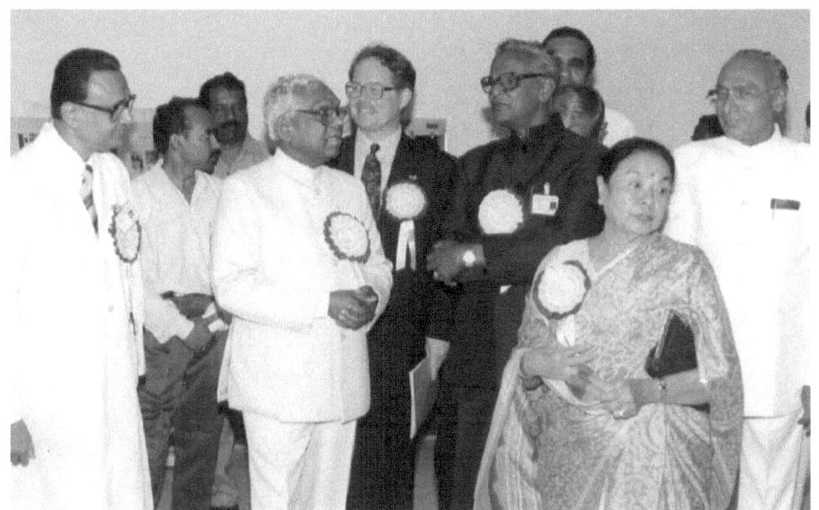

Inauguration of Linear Accelerator on 7th September 1993 by Shri KR Narayanan, the then Vice-president of India

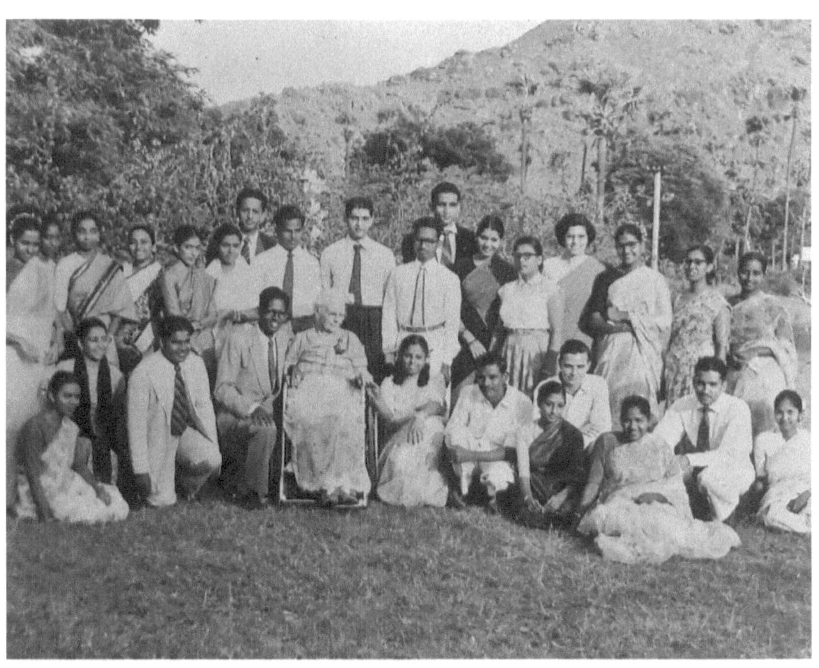

1955 Batch of medical students at 'tree planting' ceremony with Aunt Ida in 1959

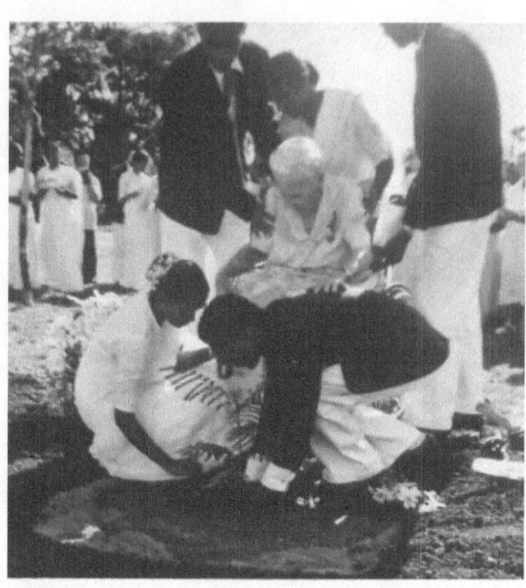

Two final year students –Nalini Banwar and Paul Premsagar– planting a tree on College Day 1959; Dr. Mathan assisting Aunt Ida who is supervising them

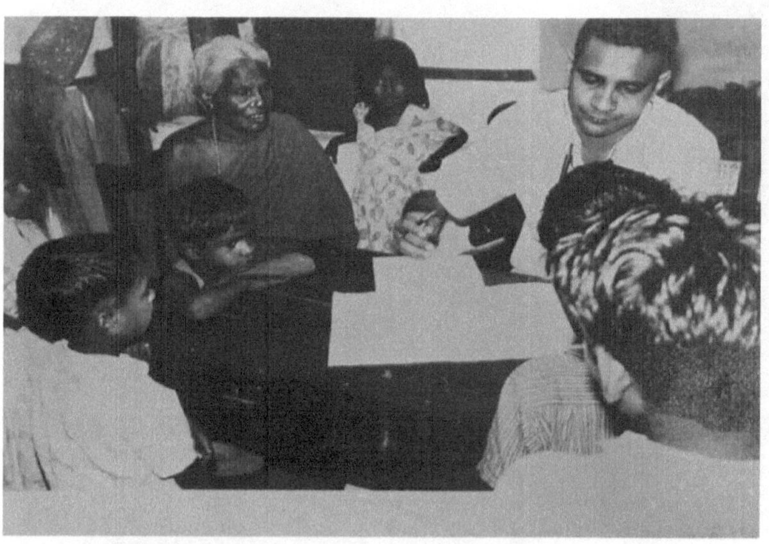

Dr Mathan at the Kaniyambadi Clinic.

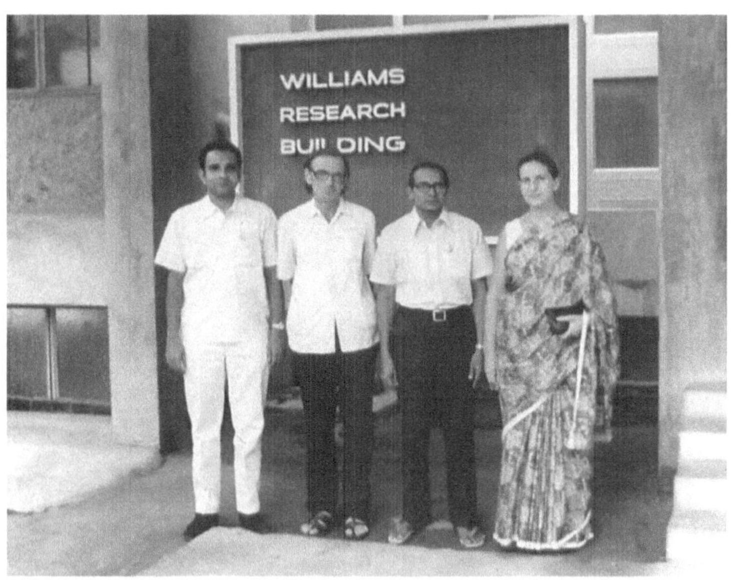

*(left to right) Dr. VI Mathan,
Dr. Selwyn Baker, Dr. AN Radhakrishnan and Mrs. Betty Baker*

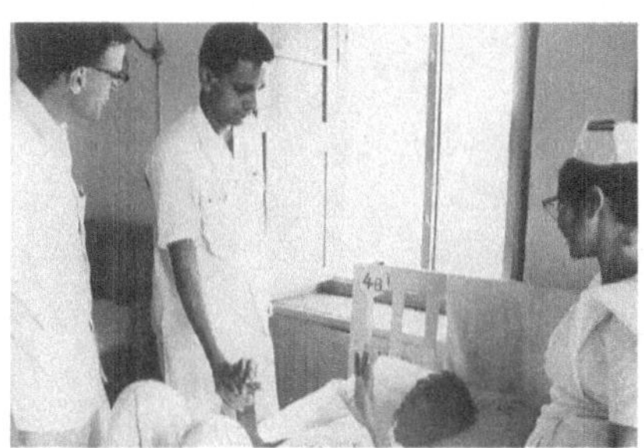

*Dr. SJ Baker (left) and Dr. Mathan
(holding the patient's hand) in W
ward*

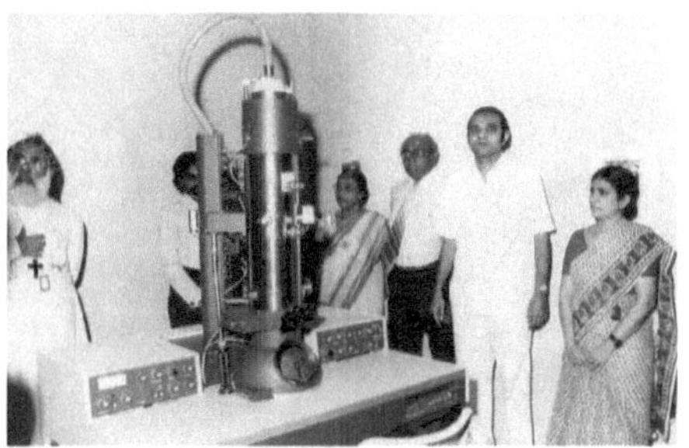

*Inauguration of the
Electronmicroscope; a grant from
the Wellcome Trust to Dr. Minnie
Mathan (extreme right, with Dr.
Mathan on her right)*

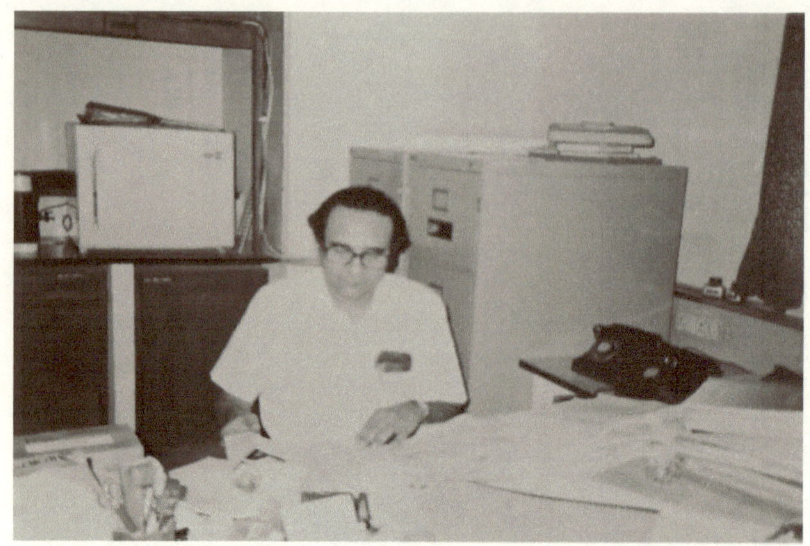

Dr Mathan at his office in the Williams Building

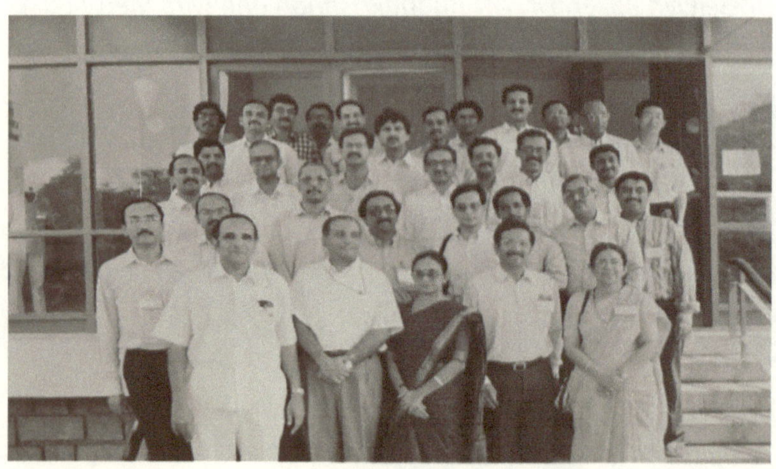

Dr Mathan with his Gastroenterology Team, 1997.

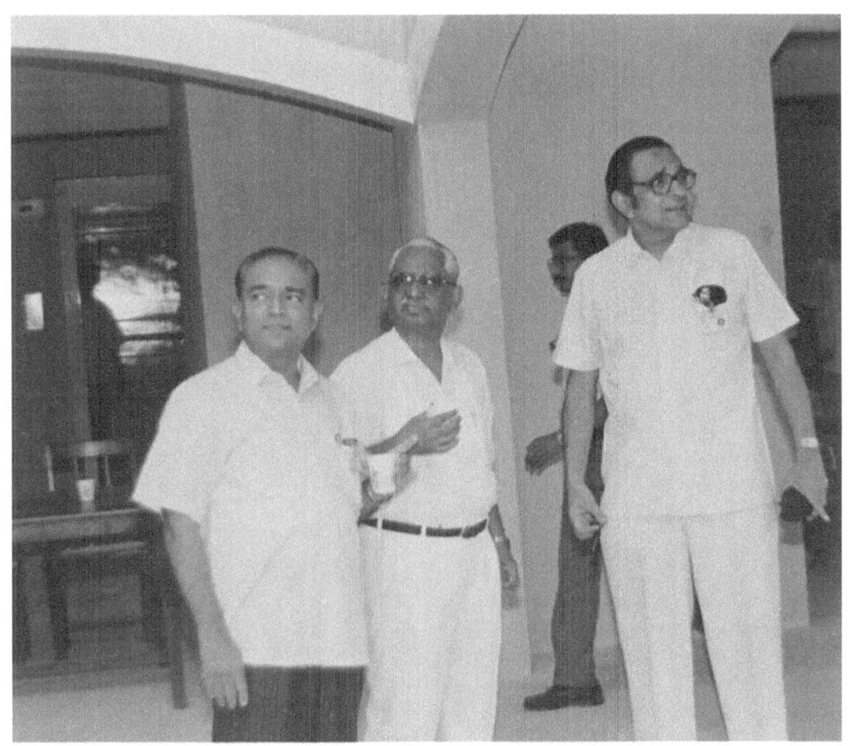

*Dr Mathan with Additional Deputy Director
Dr Kanagasabapathy and General Superintendant
Dr Jasper Daniel.*

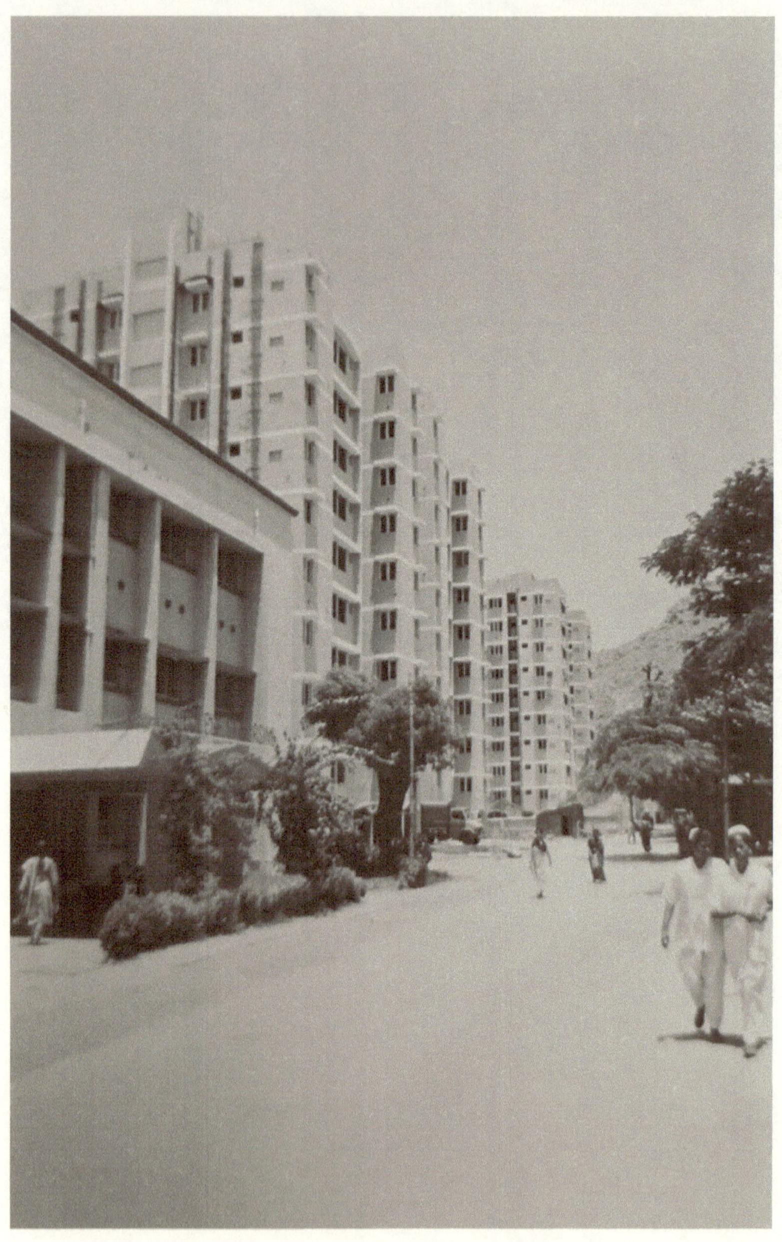

*Multi Storied Staff Quarters in
Jubilee Grounds, 1997.*

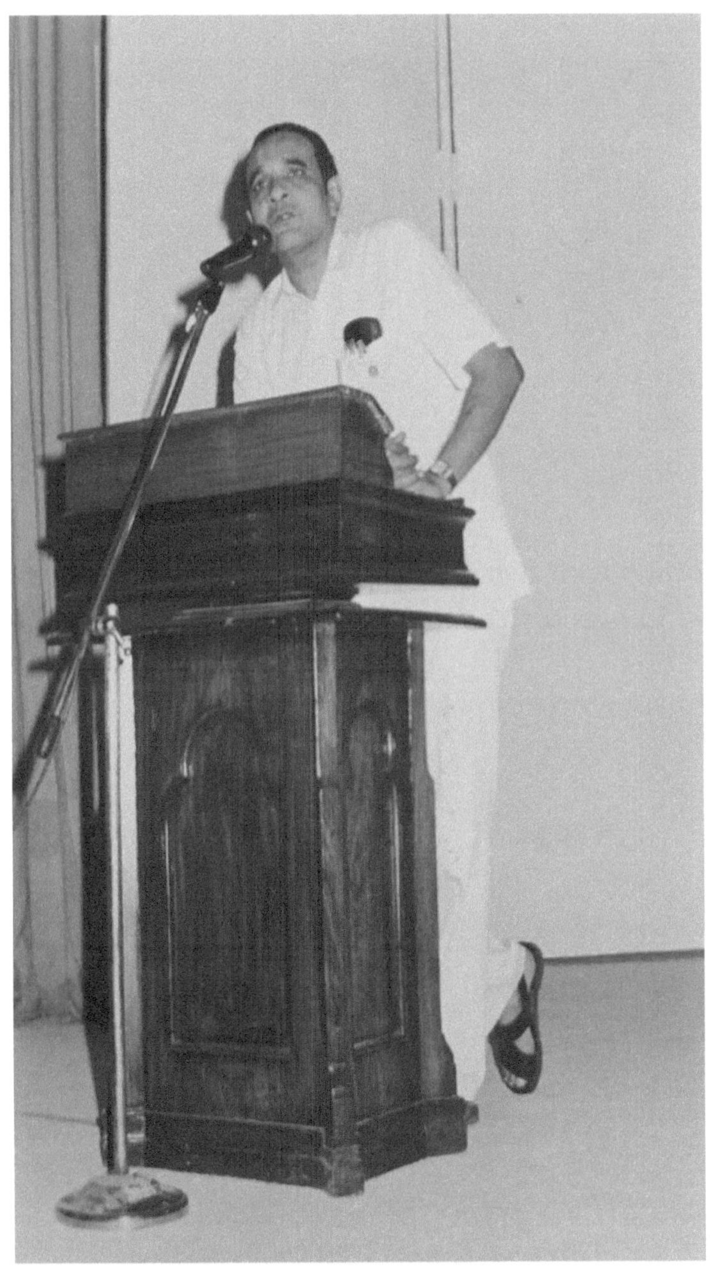

Farewell speech of Dr Mathan.

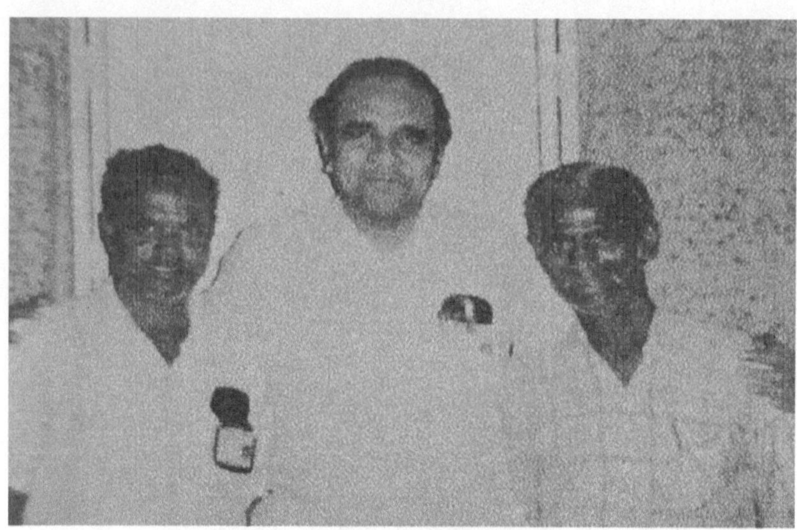

Dr. Mathan with two members of the General Service Board, Mr. Samvel (extreme right) and Mr. David Asirvadam

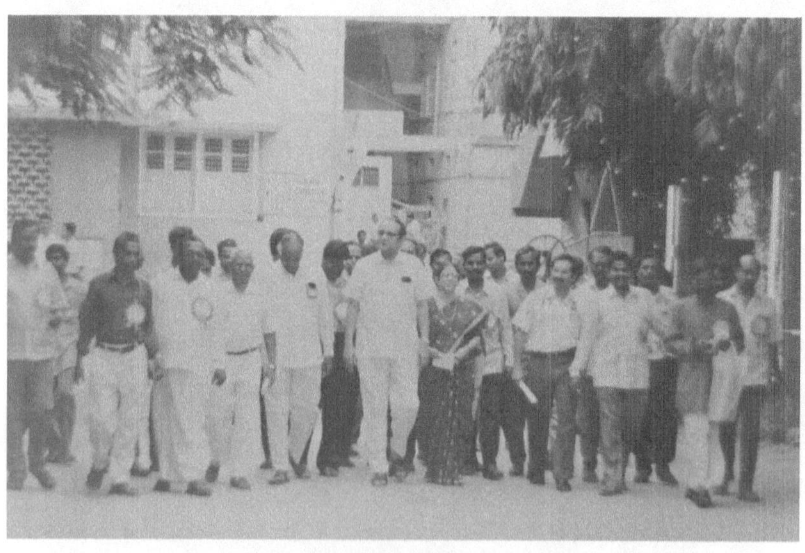

Farewell Function of Dr Mathan by general service board

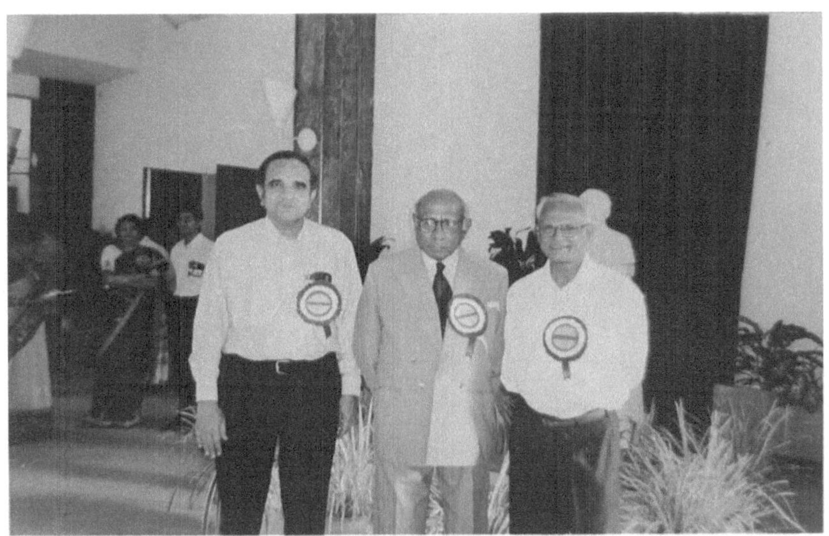

Dr Mathan with former Directors Dr LBM Joseph and Dr B M Pulimood

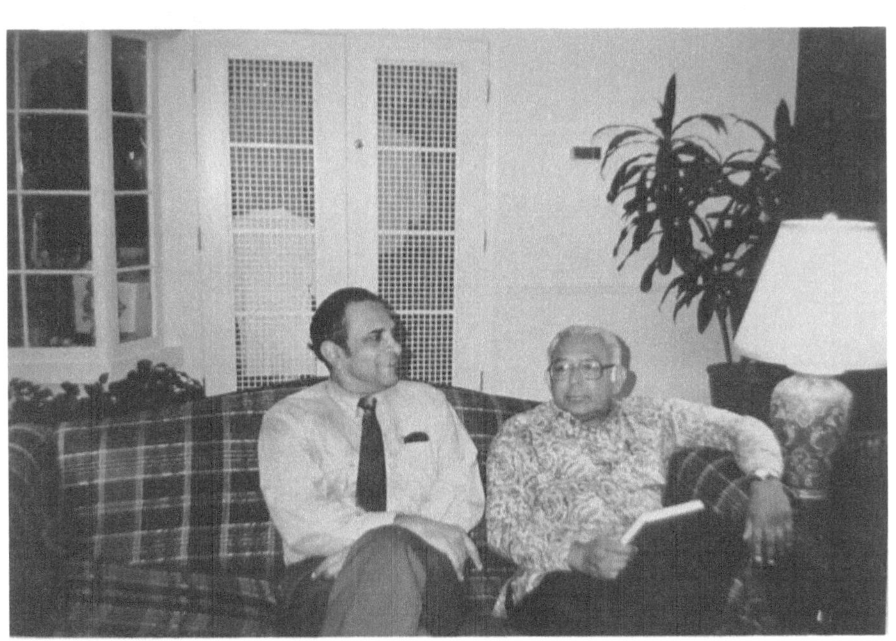

Dr Mathan with his batchmate and best friend Dr Mani M Mani.

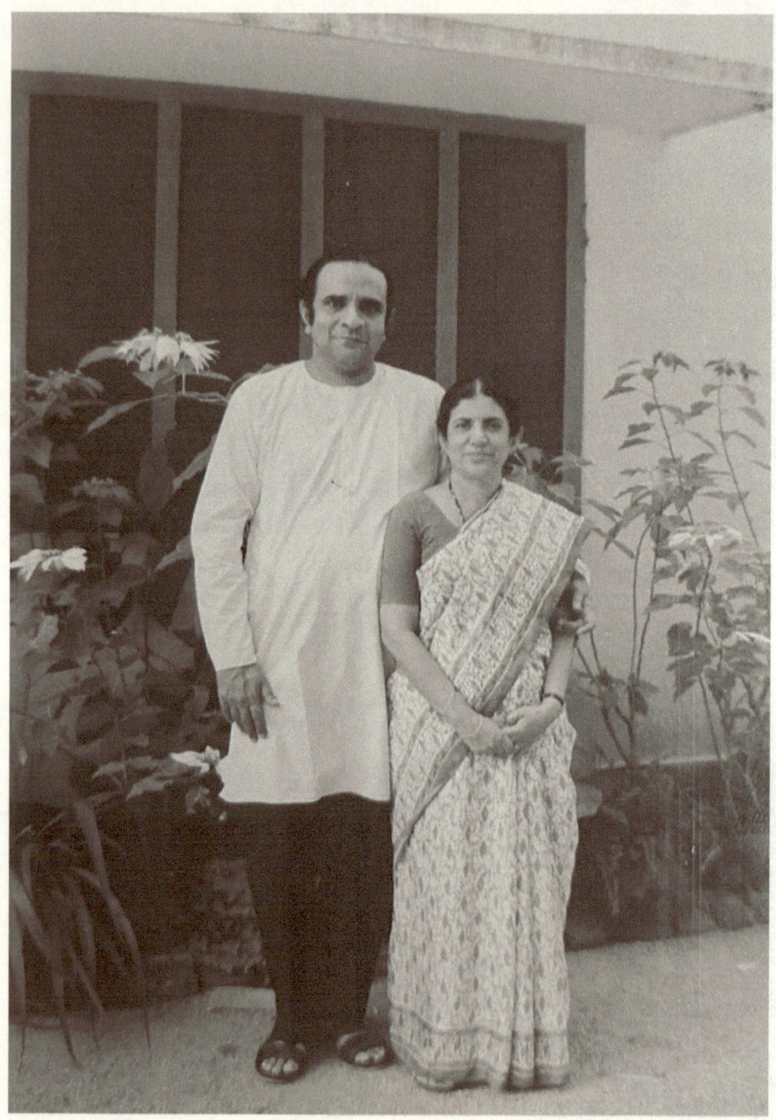

Dr. Mathan and his wife Dr. Minnie Mathan at their residence in the Vellore campus.

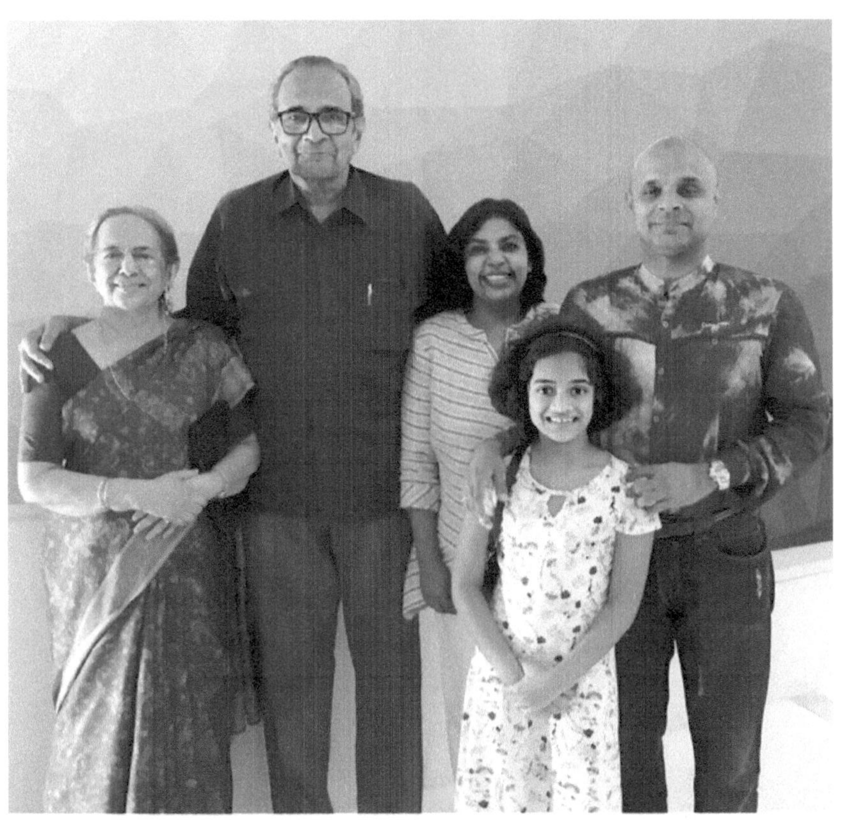

The family photograph: Dr Mathan, Mrs. Minnie Mathan, Daughter Anila Vurgese, Son-in-Law Anand Vurgese, and Grand Daughter Annika Vurgese